DIET FOR WOMEN OVER FORTY

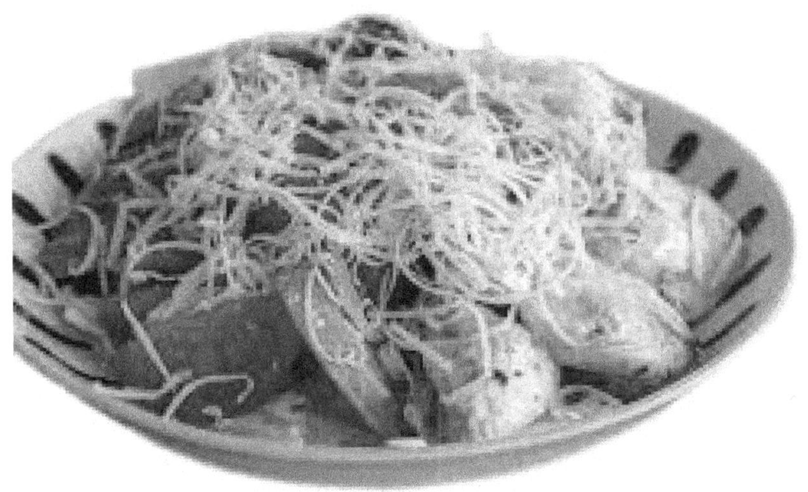

Crafting a Bodybuilding Diet for Women Over 40

Isabelle Hartley

i

OTHER BOOKS BY THIS AUTHOR

1. RECIPES FOR LOW BLOOD CHOLESTEROL
2. ATKINS DIET RECIPES COOKBOOK
3. CARDIAC DISEASE DIET COOKBOOK
4. CELIAC DISEASE RECIPES COOKBOOK
5. JUICING RECIPES FOR CANCER
6. LOW SUGAR DIET GUIDE FOR BEGINNERS

TABLE OF CONTENTS

Introduction

In the realm of fitness and well-being, the pursuit of a balanced and effective diet is paramount, and this holds especially true for women embarking on the journey of bodybuilding beyond the age of 40. As the body undergoes various changes with age, the approach to nutrition becomes a nuanced and personalized endeavor. This introduction sets the stage for understanding the unique considerations, challenges, and opportunities that come with crafting a bodybuilding diet tailored to the needs of women over 40.

Embracing a New Chapter

Entering the fifth decade of life signifies a period of change and adaptation for many women. The metabolism undergoes shifts, hormonal fluctuations become more pronounced, and the body may respond differently to diet and exercise compared to earlier years. Despite these changes, the aspiration for a healthy and strong physique remains a compelling goal.

The realm of bodybuilding provides a holistic approach to fitness, emphasizing strength, endurance, and muscle development. For women over 40, this journey is not just about aesthetics but also about cultivating resilience, maintaining bone density, and promoting overall well-being. Crafting an effective bodybuilding diet becomes a cornerstone in achieving these objectives.

Understanding Unique Needs

Women over 40 have distinct nutritional needs that demand careful consideration. One of the primary factors is the decline in muscle mass and bone density that naturally occurs with age. Adequate protein intake becomes crucial to support muscle maintenance and growth. Beyond protein, the role of carbohydrates and essential fats takes on added significance in providing sustained energy and supporting various physiological functions.

Moreover, the hormonal landscape undergoes significant changes, particularly during menopause. Fluctuations in estrogen levels can influence body composition, metabolism, and energy levels. Crafting a diet that addresses these hormonal shifts becomes pivotal in optimizing performance and mitigating potential challenges.

Individual Goals and Health Status

No two individuals are alike, and this axiom holds true when formulating a bodybuilding diet. Before diving into the intricacies of macronutrient ratios and meal timing, it's essential to conduct a thorough assessment of individual goals and health status. Factors such as existing medical conditions, dietary restrictions, and fitness objectives play a pivotal role in tailoring a diet that is not only effective but also sustainable.

Some women may pursue bodybuilding with a focus on strength training, while others may emphasize endurance or a combination of both. Understanding these goals allows for a more precise alignment of nutritional strategies to meet the unique demands of each individual.

The Role of Key Nutrients

Protein Requirements

Protein stands as the cornerstone of any bodybuilding diet, and for women over 40, its significance amplifies.

Adequate protein intake supports muscle protein synthesis, aids in recovery, and helps offset the natural decline in muscle mass associated with aging. While recommendations may vary, a general guideline is to aim for a protein intake of 1.2 to 2.2 grams per kilogram of body weight, depending on individual goals and activity levels.

Importance of Carbohydrates

Carbohydrates serve as a primary energy source, especially during intense workouts. For women over 40, incorporating complex carbohydrates into the diet provides sustained energy, helps regulate blood sugar levels, and supports cognitive function. Whole grains, fruits, and vegetables are excellent sources of complex carbohydrates that contribute to overall health and well-being.

Essential Fats

Contrary to outdated beliefs, fats are an essential component of a well-rounded bodybuilding diet. Omega-3 and omega-6 fatty acids play vital roles in hormone production, joint health, and cognitive function. Including sources of healthy fats such as avocados, nuts, seeds, and fatty fish contributes to the overall balance of the diet.

Meal Planning Strategies

With an understanding of key nutrients, the next step in crafting a bodybuilding diet involves strategic meal planning. This encompasses considerations of portion control, meal frequency, and the timing of meals to optimize nutrient absorption and energy utilization.

Portion Control

While the total caloric intake is a fundamental aspect of any diet, portion control becomes particularly relevant for women over 40. As metabolism may experience a natural slowdown, being mindful of portion sizes helps manage caloric intake and supports weight management goals. This doesn't imply drastic restriction but emphasizes the importance of balance and moderation.

Meal Frequency

The traditional three-meals-a-day approach may not be the most optimal for everyone, especially in the context of bodybuilding. Distributing caloric intake across multiple meals throughout the day helps maintain energy levels, supports muscle protein synthesis, and prevents overeating in a single sitting. Smaller, frequent meals contribute to a more sustained release of energy, supporting both daily activities and intense training sessions.

Timing of Meals

Timing plays a crucial role in maximizing the benefits of nutrition. Pre- and post-workout meals take center stage, providing the body with the necessary fuel before exertion and aiding recovery afterward. Ensuring a balance of macronutrients in these meals supports performance and enhances the body's ability to adapt to the demands of exercise.

Hydration for Optimal Performance

While often overlooked, hydration is a cornerstone of effective bodybuilding nutrition. Adequate water intake is vital for nutrient transport, temperature regulation, and overall cellular function. For women over 40, maintaining optimal hydration becomes even more critical, as aging can impact the body's thirst mechanism. Consistent and mindful hydration supports energy levels, cognitive function, and recovery.

Supplements for Women Over 40

While a well-balanced diet should ideally provide all the necessary nutrients, certain supplements can complement the nutritional intake, especially for women over 40. Common considerations include:

- Multivitamins: Ensuring a broad spectrum of essential vitamins and minerals.
- Calcium and Vitamin D: Supporting bone health, particularly relevant during and after menopause.
- Omega-3 Fatty Acids: Enhancing cardiovascular health and supporting joint function.

Supplemental choices should align with individual needs and be incorporated judiciously to fill potential nutritional gaps.

Balancing Hormones Through Nutrition

The hormonal changes that accompany aging, particularly during menopause, present unique challenges and opportunities in crafting a bodybuilding diet. Nutrition can play a pivotal role in supporting hormonal balance and mitigating potential disruptions.

Phytoestrogens

Incorporating phytoestrogen-rich foods such as soy, flaxseeds, and legumes may provide a natural source of estrogen-like compounds. While research on the efficacy of phytoestrogens is ongoing, some studies suggest potential benefits in managing certain symptoms associated with hormonal changes.

Nutrient-Rich Choices

Choosing nutrient-dense foods supports overall health and can positively influence hormonal balance. Antioxidant-rich fruits and vegetables, along with whole grains and lean proteins, contribute to a well-rounded and hormone-supportive diet.

Tailoring the Diet to Training Intensity

The nature and intensity of training significantly influence the nutritional requirements of a bodybuilder. Tailoring the diet to align with the demands of specific workouts enhances performance, supports recovery, and promotes overall training effectiveness.

Pre-Workout Nutrition

Fueling the body adequately before a workout is essential for optimal performance. A combination of carbohydrates and protein can provide the necessary energy and support muscle function during exercise. The timing of pre-workout meals or snacks depends on individual preferences and digestive comfort.

Post-Workout Nutrition

The post-workout period is a critical window for replenishing glycogen stores and initiating the recovery process. Consuming a combination of carbohydrates and protein within the first hour after exercise supports muscle recovery, reduces muscle soreness, and enhances the body's ability to adapt to training stress.

Recovery Nutrition and Rest Days

Recovery is an integral part of any bodybuilding journey, and nutrition plays a central role in this process. On rest days or lighter training days, adjusting nutrient intake to reflect lower energy expenditure is key. Emphasizing nutrient-dense foods supports the body's recovery mechanisms and prepares it for subsequent training sessions.

Addressing Common Challenges

Navigating the realm of bodybuilding for women over 40 comes with its set of challenges. Understanding and proactively addressing these challenges contribute to a more sustainable and enjoyable journey.

Metabolism Changes

The natural slowdown in metabolism that accompanies aging can impact weight management. While it's not an insurmountable obstacle, it necessitates a thoughtful and individualized approach to caloric intake and expenditure. Incorporating a combination of strength training and cardiovascular exercise contributes to metabolic health.

Dealing with Menopause

Menopause brings about significant hormonal shifts that can influence body composition, mood, and energy levels.

Managing symptoms through lifestyle and dietary interventions, in consultation with healthcare professionals, can enhance overall well-being during this transition.

Managing Stress

Stress, whether physiological or psychological, can influence the body's response to training and nutrition. Implementing stress-management strategies, such as mindfulness, adequate sleep, and regular physical activity, complements the efforts put into crafting a bodybuilding diet.

Creating a Sustainable and Enjoyable Diet

Sustainability is the linchpin of any successful diet. For women over 40 engaged in bodybuilding, a sustainable approach involves finding a balance between nutritional goals and personal enjoyment. Restrictive diets often lead to frustration and are challenging to maintain over the long term. Embracing a varied and enjoyable diet not only enhances adherence but also contributes to overall mental and emotional well-being.

Crafting a bodybuilding diet for women over 40 is a multifaceted endeavor that requires a nuanced understanding of individual needs, goals, and the dynamic interplay of nutrition with age-related changes. By embracing the unique opportunities presented by this phase of life and tailoring dietary strategies accordingly, women over 40 can not only achieve their bodybuilding aspirations but also foster a sustainable and fulfilling approach to lifelong health and wellness. As we delve into the intricacies of nutrient balance, meal planning, and addressing common challenges, the journey unfolds as a partnership between science, individuality, and the unwavering spirit that accompanies the pursuit of a strong and resilient physique.

Chapter 1: Needs of Women Over 40

Embarking on the journey of bodybuilding after the age of 40 necessitates a keen awareness of the unique needs that distinguish this demographic. As women transition into their fifth decade, a myriad of physiological changes unfolds, demanding a tailored approach to training and nutrition. In this exploration, we delve into the intricacies of these unique needs, acknowledging the transformative power of bodybuilding in enhancing both physical and mental well-being.

Metabolic Shifts and Body Composition Changes

One of the defining features of aging is the gradual decline in metabolic rate. For women over 40, this shift can impact body composition, making it more challenging to maintain or build lean muscle mass while managing body fat. The decrease in metabolic rate is partly attributed to a natural loss of muscle tissue, a process known as sarcopenia, which accelerates in the later stages of life.

Bodybuilding, with its emphasis on resistance training, assumes a pivotal role in counteracting this decline. By engaging in regular strength training exercises, women over 40 can stimulate muscle growth, boost metabolism, and mitigate the effects of sarcopenia. The unique needs of this demographic, therefore, call for a strategic integration of resistance training into their bodybuilding regimen to address these metabolic shifts effectively.

Hormonal Fluctuations and Menopause

The fifth decade often marks the onset of menopause, a transformative phase characterized by hormonal fluctuations, specifically a decline in estrogen levels. This hormonal shift brings about changes in body composition, metabolism, and energy regulation. Bodybuilding for women over 40 must navigate this hormonal terrain with a nuanced understanding of its implications.

Estrogen plays a crucial role in maintaining bone density, and its decline during menopause is associated with an increased risk of osteoporosis. Incorporating resistance training, particularly weight-bearing exercises, becomes essential to support bone health and minimize the risk of fractures.

Furthermore, hormonal changes can influence fat distribution, often leading to an increase in visceral fat. Bodybuilding offers a powerful intervention by promoting lean muscle development, which not only contributes to a more toned physique but also aids in managing body fat levels. Tailoring nutritional strategies to support hormonal balance, such as incorporating phytoestrogen-rich foods, becomes a valuable consideration in the bodybuilding journey for women over 40.

Joint Health and Flexibility

As the years progress, joint health becomes an increasingly important aspect of overall well-being. Women over 40 may experience a decline in joint flexibility and an increased risk of conditions such as osteoarthritis. Bodybuilding programs designed for this demographic must prioritize exercises that enhance joint mobility while minimizing impact.

Low-impact resistance training, including exercises that promote joint stability and flexibility, can be instrumental in preserving joint health. Additionally, incorporating activities like yoga or stretching routines complements bodybuilding efforts by fostering flexibility and mitigating the risk of injury.

Cognitive Well-being and Stress Management

Beyond the physical realm, bodybuilding holds profound implications for cognitive well-being and stress management, aspects that gain heightened significance for women over 40. The demands of career, family, and personal responsibilities can contribute to elevated stress levels, impacting both mental and physical health.

Engaging in regular physical activity, including bodybuilding, serves as a potent stress-management tool. Exercise triggers the release of endorphins, the body's natural mood enhancers, promoting a sense of well-being and resilience against stress. For women navigating the complexities of life over 40, bodybuilding becomes a holistic approach that nurtures both the body and the mind.

Nutrient Requirements and Dietary Considerations

The nutritional needs of women over 40 engaged in bodybuilding demand careful consideration to support optimal performance, recovery, and overall health. Key nutrients take on heightened importance as the body contends with the effects of aging and the unique challenges presented by menopause.

Protein Requirements

Protein, a cornerstone of any bodybuilding diet, assumes a central role for women over 40. Adequate protein intake supports muscle protein synthesis, aiding in the preservation and growth of lean muscle mass. The recommended protein intake for this demographic typically ranges from 1.2 to 2.2 grams per kilogram of body weight, with individual variations based on activity levels and goals.

Essential Fats

While the fear of fats has historically lingered, essential fats are crucial for hormonal balance, joint health, and overall well-being. Including sources of omega-3 fatty acids, such as fatty fish, flaxseeds, and walnuts, becomes imperative for women over 40 engaged in bodybuilding.

Micronutrients

Ensuring an ample supply of vitamins and minerals is vital, especially during menopause when hormonal fluctuations can impact nutrient absorption. Calcium and vitamin D, in particular, are critical for bone health and can be obtained through a combination of dietary sources and supplements.

Hydration

As the body's thirst mechanism may diminish with age, staying adequately hydrated becomes a conscious effort. Proper hydration is essential for nutrient transport, temperature regulation, and overall cellular function. Women over 40 engaged in bodybuilding should prioritize consistent water intake throughout the day.

Individualization and Personalization

Recognizing the diversity among women over 40 is paramount in tailoring bodybuilding approaches to individual needs. What works for one person may not be optimal for another, emphasizing the importance of personalized strategies. Factors such as fitness goals, medical history, preferences, and lifestyle constraints all play a role in shaping an effective bodybuilding plan.

Consulting with healthcare professionals, nutritionists, or certified trainers can provide valuable insights into individual requirements and potential limitations. This collaborative approach ensures that the unique needs of women over 40 are not only understood but also met with precision, fostering a sustainable and effective bodybuilding journey.

Empowerment and Resilience

In essence, bodybuilding for women over 40 is more than a physical endeavor—it is a pathway to empowerment and resilience. Embracing the unique needs of this demographic requires a holistic perspective that goes beyond sets and reps. It involves acknowledging the wisdom and experience that come with age, celebrating the body's capacity for transformation, and fostering a mindset of continual growth.

As women navigate the multifaceted landscape of bodybuilding beyond 40, they redefine societal norms and challenge preconceived notions of aging. The weights become not just a means of resistance but also symbols of strength, determination, and the unwavering spirit that accompanies the pursuit of optimal health and well-being. In understanding and catering to the unique needs of women over 40 in bodybuilding, we pave the way for a transformative journey—one that transcends the confines of age and embraces the limitless potential that resides within.

Chapter 2: Assessing Individual Goals

Embarking on a bodybuilding journey beyond the age of 40 necessitates a thoughtful and personalized approach. Central to this approach is the thorough assessment of individual goals and health status, laying the foundation for a tailored and effective bodybuilding plan. In this exploration, we delve into the importance of understanding one's unique objectives and health considerations, recognizing the diverse paths women over 40 may take in pursuit of their bodybuilding aspirations.

Setting Clear and Realistic Goals

The first step in the assessment process involves setting clear and realistic goals. Women over 40 engage in bodybuilding for a multitude of reasons, ranging from enhancing overall health to achieving specific aesthetic or performance-related objectives. Each goal requires a distinct approach, and clarity in goal-setting ensures that the subsequent steps in the bodybuilding journey align with individual aspirations.

Health and Longevity

For some, the primary goal of bodybuilding beyond 40 is to enhance overall health and promote longevity. This may involve focusing on functional fitness, improving cardiovascular health, and maintaining joint flexibility. Resistance training, tailored to individual capabilities and preferences, forms a key component in this holistic approach, aiming to foster not just muscular strength but also overall well-being.

Strength and Functional Fitness

Others may prioritize strength and functional fitness as their primary objectives. This could involve targeted resistance training to build muscle mass, increase strength, and improve performance in daily activities. The emphasis here is on enhancing the body's functional capacity, ensuring that strength gains translate into improved quality of life and increased resilience to physical challenges.

Aesthetic Goals

Aesthetic goals often drive individuals to embark on a bodybuilding journey. This may include sculpting a lean physique, enhancing muscle definition, or achieving a specific body composition. Tailoring the training program to incorporate both resistance training and cardiovascular exercises becomes crucial, along with a nuanced approach to nutrition to support fat loss or muscle gain, depending on individual goals.

Performance and Athletic Endeavors

Some women over 40 may be drawn to bodybuilding for the challenge of pursuing athletic endeavors. This could involve participating in competitions, events, or simply pushing personal boundaries in terms of strength and endurance. The training focus here extends beyond aesthetics to performance optimization, requiring specialized programming to enhance specific athletic attributes.

Assessing Health Status

Simultaneously, a comprehensive assessment of health status is imperative before embarking on a bodybuilding journey. Understanding the individual's current physical condition, any pre-existing medical conditions, and potential limitations ensures that the chosen approach is both safe and effective. Key aspects of health assessment include:

Medical History

A thorough review of medical history provides insights into any existing health conditions, past injuries, or surgeries. This information guides the development of a bodybuilding plan that accommodates individual health considerations.

Physical Fitness

Assessing baseline physical fitness involves evaluating cardiovascular health, muscular strength, flexibility, and body composition. This may include tests such as cardiovascular endurance assessments, strength testing, and body fat measurements. Understanding where an individual stands in terms of fitness establishes a starting point for tailored programming.

Mobility and Joint Health

Given the potential changes in joint health and flexibility that accompany aging, a specific focus on assessing mobility and joint function is crucial. Identifying any limitations or areas of concern allows for the incorporation of exercises and strategies that promote joint health and flexibility.

Hormonal and Metabolic Profile

For women over 40, hormonal changes, particularly during menopause, can influence body composition and metabolism. Consulting with healthcare professionals to assess hormonal and metabolic profiles provides valuable information for tailoring nutritional strategies and optimizing training approaches.

Lifestyle Considerations

Taking into account lifestyle factors such as stress levels, sleep patterns, and daily commitments is integral. Bodybuilding plans must align with the realities of an individual's life, ensuring that they are sustainable and realistic within the context of daily responsibilities and routines.

Individualized Training Programs

Armed with a clear understanding of goals and health status, the next step involves crafting individualized training programs. These programs encompass a blend of resistance training, cardiovascular exercises, and flexibility work, tailored to address the unique needs and objectives identified during the assessment phase.

Resistance Training

The cornerstone of any bodybuilding program, resistance training, assumes a central role in building and preserving lean muscle mass. For women over 40, the focus may involve a combination of compound exercises that engage multiple muscle groups simultaneously, promoting functional strength and overall muscle development. Resistance training programs should be structured to accommodate individual fitness levels, gradually progressing in intensity and complexity.

Cardiovascular Exercise

Incorporating cardiovascular exercises complements the resistance training component, contributing to overall cardiovascular health, calorie expenditure, and fat loss. The type, intensity, and duration of cardiovascular exercises can be tailored based on individual preferences and goals, whether it's steady-state cardio, high-intensity interval training (HIIT), or a combination of both.

Flexibility and Mobility Work

Given the importance of joint health and flexibility, integrating stretching routines and mobility exercises is crucial. This component of the program aims to enhance range of motion, reduce the risk of injury, and support overall joint health. Yoga or dedicated flexibility sessions can be valuable additions to the bodybuilding regimen for women over 40.

Nutrition Strategies Aligned with Goals

Nutrition serves as a cornerstone in achieving bodybuilding goals and optimizing health. Tailoring nutrition strategies to align with individual goals, energy requirements, and potential hormonal considerations is a critical aspect of the assessment process.

Caloric Intake

Balancing caloric intake with energy expenditure is fundamental to body composition goals. Whether the objective is fat loss, muscle gain, or weight maintenance, understanding individual caloric needs guides the development of a sustainable and effective nutrition plan.

Macronutrient Ratios

Adjusting macronutrient ratios based on individual goals is key. Protein intake, in particular, plays a pivotal role in supporting muscle preservation and growth. Carbohydrates and fats are manipulated based on energy requirements and individual preferences, ensuring a balanced and sustainable approach.

Micronutrient Considerations

Considering the potential impact of age-related changes on nutrient absorption, ensuring an adequate supply of vitamins and minerals is paramount. This may involve incorporating nutrient-dense foods and, if necessary, supplementation to address specific micronutrient needs.

Hydration

Optimal hydration supports overall health and performance. Assessing individual hydration needs and establishing habits that promote consistent water intake contributes to the success of the bodybuilding journey.

Monitoring and Adaptation

The assessment process is not static but dynamic, requiring ongoing monitoring and adaptation. Regular check-ins, progress assessments, and adjustments to the training and nutrition plan based on individual responses are integral components of a successful bodybuilding journey for women over 40.

Regular Check-Ins

Scheduled check-ins with healthcare professionals, trainers, or nutritionists provide opportunities to review progress, address any concerns, and make informed adjustments to the program. These check-ins contribute to a collaborative and supportive environment that enhances the overall effectiveness of the bodybuilding journey.

Periodization

Implementing a periodized approach to training involves strategically varying intensity, volume, and focus throughout the training cycles. This not only prevents plateaus but also allows for adequate recovery, minimizing the risk of overtraining and injuries.

Flexibility in Approach

Recognizing that life is dynamic, and circumstances may change, flexibility in approach is crucial. The ability to adapt the bodybuilding plan to accommodate changes in lifestyle, health status, or personal preferences ensures long-term sustainability.

Status serves as the compass guiding the bodybuilding journey for women over 40. It is a dynamic and empowering process that recognizes the uniqueness of each individual, fostering a personalized and sustainable approach to bodybuilding. By understanding and embracing individual aspirations, addressing health considerations, and crafting tailored training and nutrition plans, women over 40 embark on a transformative journey—one that transcends the confines of age and unleashes the full potential of the body and mind. In this holistic approach, the assessment becomes not just a preliminary step but a continual process that empowers and guides every facet of the bodybuilding adventure, propelling women over 40 toward their goals with confidence and resilience.

CHAPTER 3: Key Nutrients

Navigating the realms of bodybuilding for women over 40 requires a nuanced understanding of the nutritional landscape. In this exploration of "Key Nutrients for Women Over 40 in Bodybuilding," we delve into the pivotal role that specific nutrients play in supporting muscle health, hormonal balance, and overall well-being. As the body undergoes age-related changes, the significance of key nutrients such as protein, carbohydrates, and essential fats takes center stage. This concise guide aims to shed light on the unique nutritional needs of women over 40 engaged in bodybuilding, offering insights into optimizing dietary choices to fuel strength, promote recovery, and foster resilience in the pursuit of a strong and vibrant physique.

Protein Requirements

Protein stands as the cornerstone of any effective bodybuilding regimen, and for women navigating the dynamic landscape beyond 40, its significance becomes even more pronounced. Understanding and meeting specific protein requirements is pivotal for preserving and building lean muscle mass, supporting recovery, and addressing the age-related changes that impact the body's composition.

Preserving Lean Muscle Mass

As women age, there is a natural decline in muscle mass, a phenomenon known as sarcopenia. This decline can be accelerated by factors such as hormonal changes, sedentary lifestyles, and inadequate nutrition. Protein intake emerges as a powerful countermeasure, stimulating muscle protein synthesis and offsetting the natural loss of muscle tissue. For women over 40 engaged in bodybuilding, prioritizing protein becomes a strategic approach to preserve and enhance lean muscle mass.

Setting Protein Intake Guidelines

The general guideline for protein intake often hovers between 1.2 to 2.2 grams per kilogram of body weight, with individual variations based on factors such as activity level, training intensity, and overall health goals. Women over 40 pursuing bodybuilding goals may lean towards the higher end of this spectrum, especially if their focus is on building muscle or optimizing body composition.

Supporting Recovery and Adaptation

Effective recovery is paramount in any bodybuilding journey, and protein plays a pivotal role in this process. Post-exercise, the body's demand for amino acids, the building blocks of proteins, peaks. Adequate protein intake supports muscle recovery, reduces muscle soreness, and enhances the body's ability to adapt to the stress of training. For women over 40, whose bodies may require additional support in the recovery process, a strategic emphasis on protein becomes instrumental.

Optimizing Meal Timing

Beyond total protein intake, the timing of protein consumption is a key consideration. Distributing protein intake evenly across meals, with a focus on pre- and post-workout nutrition, enhances the body's utilization of amino acids for muscle repair and growth. This strategic approach not only supports immediate recovery but also contributes to sustained muscle protein synthesis throughout the day.

Sources of High-Quality Protein

Choosing high-quality protein sources is essential for meeting nutrient needs effectively. Lean meats, poultry, fish, eggs, dairy products, legumes, and plant-based protein sources such as tofu and quinoa offer a diverse array of options. For women over 40, incorporating a mix of these sources ensures a comprehensive intake of essential amino acids, fostering optimal muscle health.

Addressing Specific Goals

Protein requirements can be further tailored based on individual goals. Women focused on fat loss may benefit from a slightly higher protein intake to support satiety and preserve lean muscle mass during caloric deficits. Those emphasizing muscle gain might aim for the higher end of the recommended range to provide the building blocks necessary for hypertrophy.

Considerations for Hormonal Changes

Hormonal shifts, particularly during menopause, can influence protein metabolism. Ensuring adequate protein intake becomes even more critical during this phase to offset potential changes in muscle mass and metabolic rate. Customizing protein strategies to align with hormonal fluctuations contributes to the overall effectiveness of a bodybuilding plan for women over 40.

In the realm of bodybuilding for women over 40, protein stands as a pillar of strength and resilience. It not only preserves and builds lean muscle mass but also supports recovery, addresses age-related changes, and contributes to the overall success of the bodybuilding journey. Strategic attention to protein intake, considering individual goals, timing, and sources, empowers women over 40 to unlock the full potential of their bodies, fostering a strong and vibrant approach to lifelong health and fitness.

Importance of Carbohydrates

In the intricate tapestry of bodybuilding for women over 40, the role of carbohydrates takes center stage as a vital fuel source for energy, endurance, and overall performance. Understanding the importance of carbohydrates and strategically incorporating them into the nutritional plan is key to optimizing training, promoting recovery, and navigating the unique considerations that accompany this phase of life.

Sustained Energy for Workouts

Carbohydrates serve as the primary source of energy for the body, especially during high-intensity workouts. For women over 40 engaged in bodybuilding, where endurance and sustained energy are paramount, ensuring an adequate intake of carbohydrates becomes essential. Whole grains, fruits, and vegetables offer complex carbohydrates that provide a steady release of energy, supporting both resistance training and cardiovascular exercises.

Blood Sugar Regulation

The intricate dance of blood sugar levels becomes particularly relevant for women over 40, especially considering the potential impact of hormonal changes. Complex carbohydrates, rich in fiber, contribute to stable blood sugar levels, preventing sharp spikes and crashes. This not only supports energy levels during workouts but also helps maintain focus and cognitive function throughout the day.

Supporting Hormonal Balance

Carbohydrates play a role in influencing hormonal balance, which is crucial for women navigating the hormonal fluctuations associated with menopause. Optimal carbohydrate intake contributes to the regulation of insulin, cortisol, and other hormones, positively impacting metabolism and overall hormonal harmony. Balancing macronutrients, including carbohydrates, becomes a strategic component of managing hormonal changes effectively.

Replenishing Glycogen Stores

Intense workouts deplete glycogen stores, the body's stored form of carbohydrates. Adequate carbohydrate intake in the post-workout period becomes instrumental in replenishing glycogen stores, facilitating muscle recovery, and preparing the body for subsequent training sessions. This strategic approach contributes to improved endurance and helps stave off fatigue during prolonged or high-intensity workouts.

Individualized Carbohydrate Needs

While carbohydrates are a crucial component, the specific carbohydrate needs vary among individuals based on factors such as activity level, training intensity, and metabolic rate. Customizing carbohydrate intake to align with individual goals and energy requirements ensures that women over 40 receive the right amount of fuel to support their bodybuilding endeavors.

Timing and Distribution

Strategic timing and distribution of carbohydrates throughout the day contribute to optimized energy utilization and performance. Pre-workout meals or snacks with a balance of carbohydrates and protein provide a fuel source for upcoming exertion. Post-workout meals that include carbohydrates support glycogen replenishment and muscle recovery. Distributing carbohydrates evenly across meals helps maintain energy levels and supports metabolic health.

Choosing Nutrient-Dense Sources

Incorporating nutrient-dense carbohydrate sources is paramount for overall health. Whole grains, fruits, vegetables, and legumes not only provide carbohydrates but also deliver essential vitamins, minerals, and fiber. These foods contribute to satiety, digestive health, and a well-rounded nutritional profile, aligning with the holistic approach to bodybuilding for women over 40.

Adapting to Individual Goals

Carbohydrate intake can be adapted based on individual goals. Those focusing on fat loss may benefit from adjusting carbohydrate intake to create a moderate caloric deficit, while individuals aiming for muscle gain might strategically increase carbohydrate intake to support energy needs and muscle growth. This personalized approach ensures that carbohydrates align with specific body composition objectives.

In the nuanced realm of bodybuilding for women over 40, carbohydrates emerge as the engine of progress, fueling workouts, supporting hormonal balance, and contributing to overall vitality. Recognizing the importance of carbohydrates and tailoring their intake to individual needs empowers women over 40 to navigate the intricacies of bodybuilding with resilience and effectiveness. By embracing the right balance of carbohydrates, women over 40 can unlock the energy needed to sculpt a strong, vibrant, and enduring physique.

Essential Fats

In the mosaic of nutritional considerations for women over 40 in bodybuilding, the spotlight turns to essential fats, recognizing their pivotal role in hormonal balance, joint health, and overall well-being. Understanding the importance of incorporating essential fats into the dietary framework becomes crucial for optimizing performance, supporting recovery, and addressing the specific needs of this demographic.

Hormonal Balance and Women's Health

Essential fats, including omega-3 and omega-6 fatty acids, play a critical role in hormone production and regulation. For women over 40, who often contend with hormonal changes, ensuring an adequate intake of essential fats becomes instrumental in promoting hormonal balance. These fats contribute to the production of hormones that influence metabolism, mood, and overall women's health, especially during phases like perimenopause and menopause.

Supporting Joint Health and Mobility

As women age, joint health becomes a paramount consideration in any fitness journey. Essential fats showcase their importance by contributing to joint lubrication and reducing inflammation. Incorporating sources of omega-3 fatty acids, such as fatty fish, flaxseeds, and walnuts, can be particularly beneficial. These fats not only support joint health but also enhance overall mobility, a crucial aspect for women over 40 engaging in bodybuilding.

Cognitive Function and Brain Health

The benefits of essential fats extend beyond the physical realm, encompassing cognitive function and brain health. Omega-3 fatty acids, in particular, are known for their role in supporting brain function, memory, and overall cognitive well-being. As women navigate the multifaceted demands of daily life, including the intricacies of bodybuilding, prioritizing essential fats contributes to mental sharpness and resilience.

Balancing Omega-3 and Omega-6 Ratios

While both omega-3 and omega-6 fatty acids are essential, maintaining a balanced ratio between them is key. Western diets often tip the balance in favor of omega-6 fatty acids, which are abundant in processed foods and certain vegetable oils. Actively incorporating sources of omega-3s helps restore balance, contributing to anti-inflammatory effects and overall health. Balancing these ratios is particularly relevant for women over 40, given the potential impact on inflammation and age-related health considerations.

Sources of Essential Fats

Ensuring a diverse array of food sources rich in essential fats is essential for meeting nutritional needs. Fatty fish such as salmon and trout, flaxseeds, chia seeds, walnuts, and avocados are excellent choices. Incorporating these foods into the diet provides a comprehensive profile of essential fats along with additional nutrients that contribute to overall health.

Impact on Cardiovascular Health

The influence of essential fats on cardiovascular health is a critical consideration, especially as women age. Omega-3 fatty acids contribute to heart health by reducing blood pressure, improving lipid profiles, and supporting overall cardiovascular function. Given that heart health becomes increasingly relevant with age, prioritizing essential fats aligns with a holistic approach to well-being for women over 40.

Caloric Density and Moderation

While essential fats offer a myriad of benefits, it's crucial to be mindful of their caloric density. Fats are energy-dense, and moderation is key, especially for those with specific body composition goals. Integrating these fats into a well-balanced diet ensures that the benefits are reaped without compromising overall caloric balance.

Individualized Approach to Essential Fats

Recognizing the individuality of dietary preferences and needs, an individualized approach to essential fats is imperative. Some women may opt for plant-based sources, while others may include fish or omega-3 supplements. Consulting with healthcare professionals or nutritionists aids in tailoring an approach that aligns with individual goals and health considerations.

In the realm of bodybuilding for women over 40, essential fats emerge as pillars of holistic health, influencing hormonal balance, joint health, cognitive function, and cardiovascular well-being. Understanding their significance and integrating them into the dietary landscape empowers women over 40 to navigate the intricacies of bodybuilding with resilience and vigor. By embracing the multifaceted benefits of essential fats, women over 40 can fortify their bodies, nurture their minds, and embark on a bodybuilding journey that transcends the physical to encompass the full spectrum of well-being.

CHAPTER 4: Meal Planning Strategies

Embarking on a successful bodybuilding journey for women over 40 requires more than just dedication in the gym; it demands a meticulous approach to nutrition. In this exploration of "Meal Planning Strategies," we delve into the crucial role that thoughtful and strategic meal planning plays in optimizing performance, promoting recovery, and achieving body composition goals. Tailoring nutrition to the unique needs of women over 40 engaged in bodybuilding involves not only understanding the importance of key nutrients but also crafting a well-structured and sustainable meal plan. From supporting muscle health to addressing hormonal fluctuations, these meal planning strategies serve as a compass, guiding women over 40 toward a nourishing and effective approach to their bodybuilding aspirations.

Portion Control

Mastering portion control stands as a cornerstone of effective nutrition strategies for women over 40 engaged in bodybuilding. As the body undergoes age-related changes, understanding and implementing precise portion sizes becomes instrumental in achieving specific goals, managing energy intake, and optimizing overall health.

Precision in Macronutrient Balance

Portion control ensures a balanced intake of macronutrients—protein, carbohydrates, and fats— essential for supporting muscle health, energy levels, and hormonal balance. Dividing meals into appropriate portions allows for a balanced distribution of these macronutrients, supporting various body functions critical for bodybuilding success.

Caloric Management and Body Composition Goals

Controlling portion sizes directly impacts caloric intake, playing a pivotal role in managing body composition goals. For women over 40, who may have specific fat loss or muscle gain objectives, precise portion control enables the regulation of energy intake, contributing to the achievement of desired body composition changes.

Enhanced Nutrient Absorption

Portion control promotes optimal nutrient absorption by preventing overconsumption. It allows the body to efficiently utilize nutrients, ensuring that essential vitamins, minerals, and other micronutrients are absorbed effectively. This becomes particularly relevant for women over 40, where nutrient absorption efficiency may diminish with age.

Preventing Overeating and Promoting Satiety

Careful portioning aids in preventing overeating by providing a visual guide to appropriate serving sizes. Controlling portion sizes with nutrient-dense foods rich in fiber and protein fosters feelings of fullness and satiety, curbing excessive calorie intake and supporting weight management goals.

Strategic Meal Planning

Portion control is interlinked with strategic meal planning, where meals are designed with specific portion sizes aligned with individual goals and nutritional needs. By incorporating portion control into meal planning, women over 40 can craft well-balanced and purposeful meals that support their bodybuilding journey.

Utilizing Visual Cues

Employing visual cues, such as measuring tools, portion plates, or simply familiarizing oneself with typical serving sizes, facilitates portion control. This practice aids in developing a sense of portion sizes, empowering women over 40 to make informed and conscious choices about their food intake.

Flexibility and Adherence

While portion control is essential, flexibility in approach fosters adherence to dietary plans. It allows for occasional indulgences or adjustments based on social situations without compromising overall progress. The key lies in maintaining a balance between portion control and flexibility, ensuring sustainability in the long run.

Mindful Eating Practices

Adopting mindful eating practices complements portion control by encouraging a conscious and deliberate approach to meals. Paying attention to hunger cues, eating slowly, and savoring each bite contributes to improved portion awareness and aids in maintaining a healthy relationship with food.

In the realm of bodybuilding for women over 40, portion control emerges as a potent tool that guides nutritional choices, supports body composition goals, and fosters overall well-being. By mastering portion control, women over 40 harness the power to manage energy intake, optimize nutrient absorption, and steer their bodybuilding journey towards success. Embracing this foundational element paves the way for a nourishing, sustainable, and purposeful approach to nutrition, unlocking the true potential of the body and mind.

Meal Frequency

Meal frequency, a strategic element of nutritional planning, holds particular significance for women over 40 engaged in bodybuilding. Tailoring the timing and frequency of meals plays a vital role in supporting metabolic health, sustaining energy levels, and maximizing the benefits of resistance training.

Metabolic Boost and Energy Stability

For women over 40, whose metabolic rate may experience a natural decline, distributing caloric intake across multiple meals can provide a metabolic boost. Frequent, balanced meals contribute to sustained energy levels throughout the day, aiding in the prevention of energy slumps and supporting overall vitality.

Muscle Protein Synthesis and Recovery

Strategic meal frequency supports muscle protein synthesis, a crucial process for muscle repair and growth. Dividing daily protein intake across several meals ensures a steady supply of amino acids, promoting optimal recovery and enhancing the effects of resistance training. This becomes especially relevant for women over 40 aiming to preserve or build lean muscle mass.

Blood Sugar Regulation

Balancing meal frequency assists in maintaining stable blood sugar levels, a key consideration for women over 40 navigating hormonal changes. Regular, well-timed meals help prevent drastic fluctuations in blood sugar, contributing to improved mood, sustained focus, and overall cognitive well-being.

Appetite Regulation and Weight Management

Frequent, smaller meals support appetite regulation, preventing excessive hunger and potential overeating. This approach aids in weight management by controlling portion sizes and fostering a more mindful relationship with food. For women over 40 with specific body composition goals, strategic meal frequency aligns with effective weight management strategies.

Strategic Pre- and Post-Workout Nutrition

Tailoring meal frequency to include strategic pre- and post-workout nutrition enhances performance and recovery. Consuming a balanced meal or snack before training provides the necessary energy, while post-workout meals support glycogen replenishment and muscle repair. This targeted approach optimizes the benefits of resistance training sessions, contributing to the overall success of a bodybuilding program.

Customization Based on Lifestyle and Preferences

Adapting meal frequency to individual lifestyles and preferences ensures sustainability. Some women may thrive with three larger meals and a couple of snacks, while others may prefer a more frequent, smaller meal pattern. Customization allows for alignment with daily routines, preferences, and the practicalities of individual lifestyles.

Consideration of Total Daily Nutrient Intake

While meal frequency is a crucial consideration, the total daily nutrient intake remains paramount. Whether distributed across three meals or multiple smaller meals, achieving the required macronutrient and micronutrient intake is essential. The focus should be on meeting individual nutritional needs while optimizing meal timing for specific goals.

Hydration Throughout the Day

In addition to solid meals, hydration should be a constant consideration. Drinking water consistently throughout the day supports nutrient transport, digestion, and overall well-being. Women over 40 engaged in bodybuilding should prioritize hydration as an integral component of their meal frequency strategy.

Meal frequency emerges as a strategic ally for women over 40 pursuing excellence in bodybuilding. By optimizing the timing and distribution of meals, individuals can enhance metabolic efficiency, support muscle health, and regulate key physiological processes. Tailoring meal frequency to individual preferences and goals empowers women over 40 to navigate their bodybuilding journey with precision, fostering progress in performance, recovery, and overall well-being.

Timing of Meals

For women over 40 who are involved in bodybuilding, meal scheduling is a complex and deliberate aspect of nutrition. Nutrient timing corresponds with specific times of day to maximize energy use, assist metabolism, and improve overall training and recovery efficaciousness.

Nutrient Kickstart in the Morning

A healthy, nutrient-dense breakfast boosts metabolism and gives you the energy you need to get through the day. This breakfast, which provides the body with essential nutrients following the overnight fasting period and helps maintain sustained energy levels, sets the tone for the day for women over 40.

Thoughtful Fueling Before Exercise

Eating at a deliberate time before working out guarantees that energy will be available for exercising. Eating a healthy meal or snack one to two hours before to doing out provide the energy needed for peak performance. When it comes to women over 40 who want to get the most out of resistance training, this practice becomes extremely important.

Nutrient Replenishment After Exercise

A crucial time for nutrition replenishment, especially for muscle healing, is just after a workout. Within the first 30 to 60 minutes following exercise, consuming a combination of carbohydrates and protein promotes muscle protein synthesis, glycogen resupply, and general recovery. Resistance training for women over 40 is more successful when done with this customized method.

Stabilizing Nutrient Consumption During the Day

Eating meals and snacks at equal intervals guarantees a steady supply of nutrients and energy all day long. This strategy enhances metabolic function, encourages fullness, and helps control blood sugar levels in women over 40, all of which help with weight management and general well-being.

Late Night Snacks and Recuperation

Including a nutritious dinner is critical for promoting healing and supplying the nutrients needed for overnight healing. Saturating the body with a range of veggies, lean protein, and healthy fats during the evening meal aids in muscle repair and primes the body for the overnight fast.

Conscious After-Dark Snacking

Snacks consumed after midnight, if selected carefully, can help achieve certain objectives. Choosing low-calorie, high-protein foods can help control appetite and encourage muscle repair throughout the course of the night. But it's important to pay attention to both your total calorie consumption and your specific nutritional requirements.

Switching to Fit Your Own Schedule and Way of Life

When timing meals, it's important to take lifestyle circumstances and individual circadian rhythms into account. While some women might think that eating dinner early improves their performance, others might prefer to eat later. Timing meals according to daily schedules and preferences promotes sustainability and adherence.

Throughout the Day Hydration

Hydration should be planned into meal times to guarantee steady consumption of fluids. Sufficient water promotes healthy digestion, nutrient transfer, and general well-being. Staying hydrated throughout the day should be a top priority for bodybuilding women over 40. This includes drinking enough water before, during, and after exercises.

One more precise tool in the dietary toolbox for women over 40 who body-build is meal timing. Women over 40 can maximize energy utilization, promote muscle health, and improve the overall effectiveness of their bodybuilding activities by strategically timing meals to meet their objectives and preferences and strategically syncing their nutrient intake with crucial periods of the day. This exact timing acts as a potent stimulant for enhanced output, quicker recuperation, and steady advancement.

Chapter 5: Hydration for Optimal Performance

One of the most important components of bodybuilding performance, especially for women over 40, is hydration. Understanding the complex role of hydration becomes essential for supporting muscular function, promoting recovery, and managing the demanding demands of resistance training as the body experiences age-related changes. In this thorough investigation, we explore the various facets of hydration, from its physiological significance to useful tactics designed to empower women over 40 who are pursuing bodybuilding.

The Significance of Hydration in Physiology

1. Endurance and Muscle Function

The endurance and functionality of muscles are closely related to hydration. Muscle contractions can be hampered by dehydration, which reduces strength and endurance during exercise. For bodybuilding women over 40, staying properly hydrated is critical to preserving energy during resistance training sessions, which in turn affects performance improvements.

2. Body Temperature and Thermoregulation

Effective thermoregulation is essential for bodybuilding success. Maintaining adequate hydration helps the body release heat produced during physical activity, avoiding overheating and heat-related problems. The body's capacity to control temperature during resistance training and cardiovascular exercises is supported by keeping appropriate hydration, especially for women over 40 who may undergo changes in their thermoregulatory processes.

3. Flexibility and Joint Lubrication

Hydration is essential for maintaining the flexibility and health of joints by lubricating them. In order to avoid stiffness and discomfort, it is important for women over 40 to keep well-hydrated as they may experience age-related changes in joint function. Good fluid balance promotes increased joint mobility, which is essential for performing activities correctly and reducing the chance of injury.

4. Transport and Recovery of Nutrients

Staying properly hydrated makes it easier for nutrients to be transported throughout the body, which helps supply the components needed for muscle growth and healing. Recuperation is a critical component of success for bodybuilding women over 40. Staying properly hydrated aids in the body's ability to use nutrients from meals and supplements, which speeds up the healing process.

Hydration Techniques for Female Bodybuilders Over 40

1. Customized Hydration Requirements

Understanding personal hydration requirements is essential. The amount of fluid needed depends on a number of factors, including body weight, activity level, climate, and general health. Seeking advice from medical specialists or trained dietitians can offer tailored perspectives, guaranteeing that hydration tactics correspond with personal traits and objectives.

2. Drinking the Same Amount of Water All Day

Drinking water consistently is essential to maintaining proper hydration. Instead than consuming significant amounts of water at certain times of the day, women over 40 should strive for a consistent daily intake. This method promotes general fluid balance and helps avoid dehydration.

3. Hydration Before Exercise

Hydrating strategically before a workout is essential for maximizing results. Drinking water before working out guarantees that the body is well hydrated when the training begins. This exercise promotes endurance, delays the onset of weariness, and facilitates the best possible function of the muscles.

4. Hydration During Exercise

It's important to stay hydrated when working out, especially if the activity is lengthy or vigorous. Regular water consumption promotes fluid balance, guards against dehydration, and improves overall exercise performance. The right hydration plan for an exercise regimen must take the weather, including temperature and humidity, into account.

5. Equilibrium Electrolyte

Hydration is greatly aided by electrolytes such as magnesium, potassium, and salt. Electrolyte-rich drinks or supplements may be beneficial for bodybuilding women over 40, especially when there is a lot of perspiration. Maintaining an electrolyte balance promotes appropriate fluid retention and reduces the possibility of imbalances.

6. Rehydrating After Exercise

Rehydrating after a workout is essential to the healing process. Drinking fluids that include electrolytes in addition to water can help restore nutrients lost during exercise. For women over 40 who are pursuing bodybuilding ambitions, adding a source of protein to their post-workout hydration further aids muscle repair and recovery.

7. Checking the Status of Hydration

It's important to keep an eye out for indicators of dehydration, including urine color, thirst, and general wellbeing. While darker pee may suggest dehydration, light yellow urine usually shows appropriate hydration. Sustaining ideal levels of hydration involves paying attention to the body's thirst signals and modifying fluid intake appropriately.

8. Food Sources of Hydration

Not all forms of hydration come from drinks; some foods also play a big role in total fluid consumption. Eating foods high in water content, such oranges, watermelon, and celery, as well as veggies, like cucumber and celery, adds extra nutrients that are good for women over forty.

Difficulties and Points to Remember

1. Menopause-Related Issues

Hormonal fluctuations in women going through menopause over 40 can affect how much water they need. Elevated perspiration and hot flushes might increase the amount of fluid needed. For overall health, it is critical to be aware of these changes and modify hydration tactics accordingly.

2. Effects of Medication

The fluid balance and level of hydration may be affected by certain drugs. Women over 40 should be aware that some medications have adverse effects that could impact their ability to excrete or retain water. Getting advice from medical experts makes it easier to modify hydration plans for specific health issues.

3. Adjusting for dietary requirements

Dietary preferences can be accommodated by customizing hydration regimens. You can be flexible and still consume the recommended amount of fluids by adding hydrating foods to meals, infusing water with natural tastes, or drinking herbal teas.

Hydration plays a pivotal role in the complex fabric of bodybuilding for women over 40, impacting muscle function, recuperation, and overall performance. Women over 40 can navigate the shifting terrain with accuracy if they comprehend the physiological necessity of staying hydrated and put individualized methods into practice. Every element, from a regular daily intake to thoughtful pre- and post-workout hydration, supports women over 40's overall wellbeing and gives them the confidence to follow their bodybuilding goals with maximum vitality and resilience.

Chapter 6: Supplements for Women Over 40

When it comes to nutrition, bodybuilding requires a more sophisticated strategy for women who are forty years of age and older. A balanced diet is the cornerstone, but specific supplements can provide tailored assistance to meet the particular requirements and difficulties faced by women in this age range. In this thorough investigation, we examine the essential vitamins that can help women over 40 who body-build by maintaining muscle function, improving overall performance, and optimizing health.

1. Minerals and Multivitamins

Insurance for Vitality through Nutrition

As a nutritional safety net, a premium multivitamin and mineral supplement supplies vital micronutrients that can be difficult to get from diet alone. In order to guarantee a complete intake of vitamins and minerals essential for general health and wellbeing, a multivitamin is recommended for women over 40 who may have higher nutrient requirements because of age-related factors and hormonal changes.

Support for Bone Health

As women age, calcium and vitamin D, which are essential for maintaining healthy bones, become even more important. These nutrient supplements assist maintain bone density and may lower the risk of osteoporosis. Long-term skeletal health can be enhanced by a multivitamin that contains enough calcium and vitamin D, especially for women over 40 who may be more vulnerable to bone-related problems.

2. Fatty Acids Omega-3

Joint and Cardiovascular Health

For female bodybuilders over 40, omega-3 fatty acids—which are mostly present in fatty fish and some plant sources—offer a plethora of advantages. Omega-3 fatty acids provide cardiovascular benefits, but they also improve flexibility and reduce inflammation, which is good for joints. As people age, joint issues may become more common, therefore taking omega-3 supplements can help improve general joint function.

Psychological Health

Omega-3 fatty acids have a number of cognitive benefits, including maintaining brain health and function. Omega-3 supplements may improve cognitive well-being and contribute to mental sharpness for women managing the many demands of daily life, including the challenges of bodybuilding training.

3. Supplements with Protein

Recovery and Support for Muscles

Getting enough protein is essential for maintaining and gaining lean muscle mass, particularly for bodybuilding women over 40. Convenient and effective ways to satisfy increasing protein needs are protein supplements, including whey protein or plant-based solutions like pea protein. These supplements help with muscle repair and recovery, and they can be especially helpful when it's difficult to get enough protein from complete meals.

Convenience and Meal Replacement

Protein supplements can also be used as easy meal substitutes, particularly for people with hectic schedules. Having an easy-to-access protein source can help women over 40 balance their many duties while meeting their nutritional needs without sacrificing their dietary objectives.

4. Supplements with Collagen

Skin and Joint Assistance

The protein collagen, which is widely distributed in connective tissues, is essential for maintaining skin suppleness and joint function. Collagen synthesis in women naturally decreases with age, which affects joint function and ages the skin. Supplemental collagen offers a focused supply of this protein, promoting joint flexibility and maybe improving skin health.

Benefits for Hair and Nails

Supplemental collagen may help improve the condition of your hair and nails. Collagen supplements offer further help in preserving the strength and texture of hair and nails for women over 40 who may notice changes in these areas of physical health.

5. *Folic Acid*

Support for Energy Metabolism

With the creation of red blood cells and energy metabolism, vitamin B12 becomes increasingly important for women over 40. With aging, the body's capacity to absorb B12 may diminish; nonetheless, supplements can guarantee sufficient amounts. Sustaining adequate levels of B12 promotes long-lasting energy, which enhances general vitality and endurance during bodybuilding exercises.

Mood and Cognitive Function

B12 is also involved in mood management and cognitive function. B12 supplements may benefit women over 40 by promoting mental clarity and a happy mood, both of which are important for juggling the demands of daily life with an intense bodybuilding program.

6. Calcium

Antibody Assistance

The "sunshine vitamin," vitamin D, is essential for healthy immune system operation. Vitamin D supplementation becomes a proactive tool to promote immunological health for women over 40, who may face age-related alterations in immune response, particularly in conditions when sun exposure is limited.

Augmenting Bone Health

Vitamin D supports bone health by aiding in the absorption of calcium in addition to its immune-boosting properties. For women over 40, supplementing with calcium and vitamin D can be very beneficial in strengthening and resilient bones.

7. Supplements for Pre-Workout

Increased Vigor and Attention

Supplements for pre-workout that include beta-alanine, caffeine, and branched-chain amino acids (BCAAs) might help increase focus and energy levels when working out. These supplements can give busy women over 40 the extra motivation they need to maximize their training sessions and raise the caliber of their workouts overall.

Adaptogens to Reduce Stress

Adaptogens, such as ashwagandha or rhodiola, are found in some pre-workout supplements and may help with stress management. Because stress can affect recuperation and general health, adding adaptogens to pre-workout supplements can help women deal with the complex demands of everyday life.

8. Protein and Carbohydrate Supplements After Exercise

Repair of Muscle and Glycogen Resupply

Nutrition after exercise is essential for muscle repair and glycogen resupply. Taking a supplement containing a mix of protein and carbs helps to support these functions. For bodybuilding women over forty, when recuperation is crucial, post-workout nutrition maximizes the advantages of resistance training.

Time and Convenience

Supplements after exercise are convenient, particularly in situations where entire foods might not be easily accessible. The timing of nutrient consumption following exercise affects the body's capacity for recovery; therefore, post-workout supplementation should be considered a calculated part of the full nutritional regimen.

Thoughts on Supplement Utilization

1. Tailored Needs and Objectives

Individual needs and objectives should be the basis for the decision to include supplements. Getting advice from medical professionals or licensed dietitians facilitates the process of customizing supplement selections to meet individual nutritional needs, bodybuilding goals, and health concerns.

2. Utilizing Whole Foods as the Main Source

A well-balanced diet cannot be substituted by supplements. Nutrients should still mostly come from whole meals. Supplements are deliberate additions that help particular areas of performance and health and bridge any potential nutritional shortages.

3. Pure and High-quality

To guarantee purity and potency, select high-quality supplements. Using trustworthy brands or conducting independent testing gives consumers confidence in the supplement's dependability. To ensure the integrity of the product, women over 40 should give priority to taking supplements from reliable providers.

4. Tracking and Modifying

It is crucial to regularly assess total dietary intake and modify supplement use as necessary. Dietary practices, levels of physical activity, and overall health can all change and impact the requirement for supplements. Regular evaluation guarantees that supplement selections are in line with changing objectives and situations.

5. Medication Interactions and Health Considerations

People over 40 should be aware of any underlying medical issues and any drug and supplement interactions. Making educated judgments about supplement use and ensuring compatibility with unique health profiles are made possible by open discussion with healthcare practitioners.

Supplements become tactical partners in the complex world of bodybuilding for women over 40, providing focused support to maximize health, performance, and general well-being. Every supplement, from basic multivitamins to those that focus on joint health, protein requirements, and recuperation, has a distinct function in meeting the complex demands of women in this age range. Through informed decision-making, experience, and a customized approach when it comes to supplements, women over 40 can improve their bodybuilding journey and realize their potential for long-term health, resilience, and advancement.

Chapter 7: Balancing Hormones Through Nutrition

Hormonal balance becomes vital when women start bodybuilding, especially after 40, since it has a profound impact on their overall health, performance, and body composition. Nutrition is essential for balancing hormonal swings and meeting the specific requirements of women in this age range. We explore the complex relationship between hormones and diet in this in-depth guide, providing advice and tactics to help women over 40 attain hormonal balance and maximize their bodybuilding efforts.

Comprehending Hormonal Alterations in Women Over Forty

1. Menopause and Perimenopause:

For women over 40, the perimenopause and menopause represent a major hormonal shift. Changes in the levels of estrogen, progesterone, and testosterone can affect energy expenditure overall, muscle mass, and metabolism. Comprehending these modifications establishes the basis for customizing dietary approaches to bolster hormonal equilibrium.

2. Sensitivity to Insulin

As we age, our sensitivity to insulin tends to decline, which affects how our bodies metabolize carbs. Controlling insulin levels becomes essential for bodybuilding women over 40 in order to promote energy use, avoid fat storage, and maximize nutrient partitioning.

3. Control of Cortisol:

Emotional or physical stress can raise cortisol levels. Hormonal imbalances brought on by prolonged stress may have an impact on muscle preservation and metabolism. When it comes to reducing hormone swings brought on by stress, nutrition becomes an effective strategy.

4. Thyroid Activity:

Hormonal homeostasis in general depends on healthy thyroid function. Thyroid function variations in women over 40 may affect their energy and metabolism. In order to maintain proper hormonal balance and support thyroid function, nutrition is essential.

Nutritional Techniques for Hormone Equilibrium

1. Equilibrium Macronutrient Consumption:

Hormonal balance is based on achieving a balance of the macronutrients—protein, carbs, and fats. Protein is necessary for women over 40 who participate in bodybuilding as it promotes muscle health and repair. Energy comes from carbs, and hormone production is aided by good fats. Hormonal balance is supported by adjusting macronutrient ratios to each person's needs and objectives.

2. Intricate Carbohydrates for Long-Term Energy:

Including complex carbs in your diet—found in whole grains, fruits, and vegetables—supports stable blood sugar levels and offers a consistent energy source. This is especially important for women over 40 who want to control their insulin sensitivity and maximize their body's use of energy when working out for bodybuilding.

3. Nutritious Fats for Hormone Synthesis:

The synthesis of hormones is significantly influenced by healthy fats, such as monounsaturated and omega-3 fatty acids. These fats aid in the manufacture of hormones that are essential for mood regulation, metabolism, and general health. Nuts, avocados, and fatty fish are a few examples of foods that support hormonal health.

4. Diet High in Protein to Preserve Muscle:

Maintaining lean muscle mass requires consuming enough protein, particularly for women over 40 whose muscle composition is changing due to aging. Lean meats, dairy, legumes, and plant-based protein sources are examples of diets high in protein that promote muscular health and hormonal balance.

5. Antioxidants and phytonutrients:

Including a range of vibrant fruits and vegetables in your diet offers antioxidants and phytonutrients that help lower inflammation and promote general health. These substances reduce oxidative stress and encourage normal cellular activity, which supports hormonal balance.

6. Water for Enzymatic Health:

Hormone control and general health depend on getting enough water. Water aids in several metabolic processes and helps hormones move throughout the body. To maximize hormonal function, bodybuilding women over 40 should emphasis drinking plenty of water on a regular basis.

7. Fiber as a Digestive Aid:

A high-fiber diet promotes gut health by affecting the microbiome and hormone balance. Fiber helps the body get rid of extra hormones, which helps control the amount of estrogen in the body. Fruits, vegetables, legumes, and whole grains are all great sources of dietary fiber.

8. Most Important Micronutrients:

Hormonal equilibrium depends on getting enough of the important vitamins and minerals. Important micronutrients include zinc and magnesium, which are involved in several hormonal processes, and vitamin D, which affects the synthesis of hormones. Potential shortages are addressed and general hormonal health is supported by a nutrient-dense, well-rounded diet.

Dietary Strategies and Particular Hormonal Considerations

1. Balance of Estrogen:

Phytoestrogen-Rich Foods: Including foods high in phytoestrogens, like legumes, soy, and flaxseeds, may help maintain the proper balance of estrogens in the body.

- Vegetables High in Crucerity: Compounds found in broccoli, cauliflower, and kale support balance by aiding in the breakdown of estrogen.

2. Help for Progesterone:

- Vitamin B6: Progesterone synthesis is supported by foods high in vitamin B6, including fish, poultry, and bananas.

- Foods High in Magnesium: Magnesium, which is present in nuts, seeds, and leafy greens, helps maintain the balance of all hormones, including progesterone.

3. Optimization of Testosterone:

- Foods High in Zinc: The creation of testosterone requires zinc. Good sources of zinc include meat, oysters, and pumpkin seeds.

Training in Resistance: Resistance exercise enhances natural testosterone production and should be incorporated into a bodybuilding regimen.

4. Sensitivity to Insulin:

Fiber and Whole Foods: Placing a focus on whole foods high in fiber can help control insulin sensitivity. Controlling processed carbs and refined sugars helps maintain stable blood sugar levels.

- Standard Time for Meals: Timing meals consistently and distributing macronutrients in a balanced way help control the insulin response.

5. Control of Cortisol:

Adaptogenic Herbs: Adding adaptogenic herbs to a diet, such as rhodiola and ashwagandha, may help regulate cortisol levels when stress levels are high.

- Balanced Nutrition: Preventing excessive cortisol release can be achieved by eating balanced meals and avoiding severe calorie deficiencies.

6. Support for Thyroid:

Foods High in Iodine: The thyroid depends on iodine to function. Thyroid health is supported by eating foods high in iodine, such as dairy, seafood, and seaweed.

Sources of Selenium: Sunflower seeds and Brazil nuts are good sources of selenium, which is necessary for the conversion of thyroid hormone.

Hormonal Balance and Lifestyle Factors

1. Enough Sleep:

Hormonal equilibrium depends on getting a good night's sleep. Making enough sleep a priority helps to maintain growth hormone, cortisol, and general hormonal balance.

2. Habitat Control:

Hormonal balance is influenced by stress-reduction strategies that work, such as yoga, meditation, and deep breathing exercises. Women over 40 who body-build should adopt stress-reduction techniques because long-term tension might upset hormonal balance.

3. Physical Activity on a Regular Basis:

Hormonal health is enhanced by regular physical activity, which includes both cardiovascular and resistance training. Exercise improves cortisol regulation, insulin sensitivity, and hormonal balance in general.

4. Hormone Surveillance:

Hormone status can be better understood through routine health examinations that include measurements of hormone levels. Observing hormonal levels enable smart dietary and lifestyle modifications based on personal hormonal profiles.

In the complex fabric of bodybuilding for women over forty, nutritionally establishing hormonal balance becomes essential to success. Women over 40 can empower themselves to navigate the transformative journey of bodybuilding with resilience, vitality, and optimal well-being by accepting lifestyle factors that support hormonal balance, understanding the specific hormonal considerations, and putting targeted nutritional strategies into practice. Hormone balance via diet goes beyond appearances; it becomes a significant investment in overall well-being and reaching one's greatest potential.

Chapter 8: Tailoring the Diet to Training Intensity

Bodybuilding success is primarily based on the interaction between training intensity and diet, and for women over 40, this dynamic calls for a nuanced strategy. Adjusting the diet to the demands of high-intensity exercise becomes a critical factor in maximizing results, facilitating recovery, and reaching body composition objectives. In this extensive manual, we explore the nuances of matching dietary approaches to training volume, offering perceptions and useful suggestions to support women over 40 in their bodybuilding endeavors.

Understanding Women Over 40's Training Intensity

1. Thoughts on Resistance Training:

- Aging Adaptations: Maintaining or developing lean muscle mass becomes more and more important for women as they age. As a cornerstone, resistance training promotes general strength, metabolic health, and muscular health.

- Periodization: By arranging training regimens into phases with different volumes and intensities, periodization enables focused adaptations. This strategy encourages steady advancement and helps avoid plateaus.

2. Integrating Cardiovascular Exercise:

- Healthy Metabolism: Exercise that involves the heart improves metabolic health overall. Cardio exercises help women over 40 burn calories, improve cardiovascular fitness, and control their weight.

- Physical Condition: Selecting low-impact cardiovascular exercises, like cycling or swimming, can be beneficial for joint health, especially when people adjust to age-related changes.

3. Adaptability and Rehab Techniques:

Work on the Go: Exercises that combine mobility and flexibility promote joint health and range of motion. For women over 40, this becomes especially important because flexibility promotes overall health and the avoidance of injuries.

Active Recuperation: Active recovery sessions, like yoga or low-impact aerobic exercises, improve circulation, lessen muscular soreness, and facilitate recuperation in between high-intensity training sessions.

Dietary Plans Adapted to Training Level

1. Nutrition Before Exercise:

- Available Energy: Optimizing energy availability can be achieved by adjusting pre-workout diet to training intensity. A balanced lunch or snack with carbohydrates, protein, and a moderate quantity of healthy fats provides sustained energy for moderate-to-high-intensity activities.

- Aqueous: Before working out, it's important to drink enough water to ensure peak performance. Taking into account variables such as workout time and temperature aids in determining the right amount of fluid consumption.

2. Nutrition Prior to Exercise:

- Continuation of Hydration: Staying hydrated is crucial when exercising. In order to prevent dehydration during longer or high-intensity sessions, it becomes increasingly important to periodically sip water.

Electrolyte Matter to Consider: When engaging in lengthy or strenuous exercise, especially in warmer weather, it might be beneficial to restore lost minerals through perspiration by consuming electrolyte-rich beverages or supplements.

3. Nutrition After Exercise:

Replenishment of Protein and Carbohydrates: One of the most important times of day to enhance muscle recovery and replace glycogen stores is right after an exercise. Eating a mix of carbohydrates and protein speeds up these processes and encourages the best possible recovery.

- Timing Considerations: The advantages of post-workout nutrition are maximized when consumed 30 to 60 minutes after training. This timing becomes especially important for women over 40 who want to maximize the synthesis of muscular protein.

4. Modulating Energy Consumption:

- Equivalent Energy Use: Maintaining a caloric intake in line with training intensity guarantees that the body gets the fuel it needs to support exercise and recuperation. Achieving body composition goals requires modifying calorie intake according to training phases and goals.

Periodic Reassessments: Ongoing adaptation and advancement are supported by periodically reevaluating dietary requirements in light of modifications to training volume, body composition, and general health.

Considerations for Macro and Micronutrients

1. Intake of Protein:

- Preservation of Muscle: Making sure that women over 40 who bodybuild prioritize getting enough protein. Protein aids in the maintenance and regeneration of muscles, particularly during periods of more intense training.

- Property Distribution Intake: Getting your protein from meals and snacks helps ensure that you have an even supply of amino acids throughout the day. This method helps to maximize the synthesis of muscle proteins.

2. Time Scale for Carbohydrates:

- Aligning Carbohydrates with Exercise Requirements: Optimizing carbohydrate intake according to workout volume and intensity promotes efficient use of energy. On days when you engage in longer aerobic sessions or heavy resistance training, you may need to consume more carbohydrates.

Complete Food Supplies: Stressing complex carbs from entire food sources promotes general health and long-lasting energy. Including fruits, vegetables, and grains helps create a well-balanced profile of carbohydrates.

3. Nutritious Fats for Long-Term Energy:

- Moderate Fat Intake: A diet rich in healthy fats offers a concentrated source of energy. During training sessions, a moderate intake of fats from foods like avocados, almonds, and olive oil promotes sustained energy.

- When to Consume Fat: Modify

It can be advantageous to time fat ingestion according to workout intensity. For optimal nutritional utilization, consume less fat prior to exercise and include fat in meals thereafter.

4. Diet Rich in Micronutrients:

Diversity of Nutrients: A diet high in micronutrients should be prioritized because it promotes general health and performance. A wide range of vitamins and minerals are provided by a diversity of vibrant fruits and vegetables, which supports healthy physiological function.

Accomplishments as Required: Targeted micronutrient supplementation ensures that potential gaps are filled based on individual dietary patterns and demands, supporting overall well-being.

Water Management Techniques for All Training Stages

1. Hydration Every Day:

- Reliable Fluid Consumption: Drinking enough water throughout the day promotes general health and improves mental performance. Regular hydration should be a top priority for women over 40, taking their own needs and activity levels into account.

- Using Whole Foods to Hydrate: Eating meals high in water content, such fruits and vegetables, helps maintain a balanced fluid intake. This is in line with the objective of staying hydrated without turning to conventional beverage sources.

2. Hydration Before Exercise:

Vigilant Water Intake: Drinking water prior to exercise guarantees that you are fully hydrated when you start training. Customized hydration techniques are supported by modifying intake according to preferences and environmental circumstances.

3. Hydration During Exercise:

Suck-and-Swallow Method: Regular drinking while exercise is beneficial in avoiding dehydration. By taking little sips at regular intervals, the sip-and-swallow method guarantees sustained hydration without creating pain.

Electrolyte Matter to Consider: When engaging in extended or strenuous exercise, especially in warmer climates, thinking about electrolyte-rich drinks or supplements helps to preserve electrolyte balance.

4. Hydration After Exercise:

Rehydrating Priority: It is best to concentrate on rehydrating during the post-workout interval. After a workout, drinking water and eating a well-balanced meal promotes recovery and optimal hydration.

Checking the Color of Urine: Urine color monitoring is a useful method of determining one's level of hydration. Generally speaking, light yellow pee suggests sufficient hydration, however darker urine may signal a need for more fluid consumption.

Modulating Diet to Meet Training Objectives and Phases

1. Muscle Building and Bulking:

- Excess Calorie: Adopting a small calorie surplus helps meet the higher energy requirements of vigorous resistance training during bulking periods, when the objective is strength and muscle growth.

- Putting Protein Intake First: Protein consumption is still very important since it provides the amino acids required for muscle synthesis and repair. It becomes important to modify macronutrient ratios in order to promote muscle growth objectives.

2. Fat Loss and Cutting:

- Deficit in Calorie: A small calorie deficit during fat-loss cutting stages helps to achieve the objective of lowering body fat. Lean muscle mass can be maintained by modifying total calorie consumption while keeping protein intake constant.

- Strategic Carbohydrate Manipulation: By modifying carbohydrate intake in accordance with training volume and timing, fat utilization can be maximized while meeting exercise-related energy requirements.

 3. Upkeep Stages:

Caloric Balance: To maintain current body weight, maintenance phases entail balancing caloric intake with energy expenditure. During these times, optimizing the ratios of macronutrients promotes general health and performance.

Pay Attention to Nutrient Quality: Making nutrient-dense foods a priority guarantees that the body gets the necessary vitamins and minerals, promoting general health during maintenance stages.

Personalized and Frequent Evaluations

1. Personalized Method:

Self-Recognition and Tolerance: Adherence is improved when dietary plans are customized to each person's preferences and tolerances. Sustainable diet programs benefit from taking into account aspects such as digestion, dietary restrictions, and food preferences.

- Sensitivity Monitoring: Making dietary modifications is made possible by being aware of a person's specific sensitivity or intolerance to certain foods. This customized technique promotes digestive comfort and general well-being.

2. Ongoing Evaluations:

- Recovery and Performance Metrics: Keeping an eye on performance indicators, such strength increases and endurance throughout workouts, sheds light on how well diet supports high training volumes. A recovery's worth, including weariness and muscular soreness, is assessed to guide changes in dietary plans.

- Changes in Body Composition: Monitoring alterations in body composition, encompassing muscle mass and body fat percentages, facilitates the optimization of calorie consumption and macronutrient proportions. Ongoing advancement toward body composition objectives is facilitated by routine evaluations.

Consistency and Lifestyle Elements

1. Quality of Sleep:

Affect on Recuperation: Making sleep a priority is essential to promoting recovery after strenuous exercise sessions. Getting enough good quality sleep is important for hormone balance and general health.

- Regular Sleep Schedules: Keeping regular sleep schedules helps the body respond to the circadian rhythm, which maximizes the release of hormones that are essential for healing and adaptation.

 2. Habitat Control:

- Hormone Influence: It's critical to manage stress using practical methods like mindfulness, meditation, or relaxation techniques. Persistent stress can throw off hormone balance, which can affect general health and performance in the gym.

Repeated Stress-Reduction Techniques: Stress management techniques are a proven way to increase resilience and adaptability, two traits that bodybuilding women over 40 need to possess.

 3. Assistive Supplementation:

Use of Strategic Supplement: Strategic supplement integration based on personal needs promotes overall nutritional objectives. This could involve taking specific vitamin, mineral, or performance-enhancing drug supplements.

- Consistency and Quality: It is essential to guarantee the caliber and regularity of supplement consumption. Consistent evaluation of supplement selections in light of changing objectives and health-related factors ensures adherence to nutritional protocols.

Precisely matching training intensity to diet becomes a potent catalyst for body composition objectives, recuperation, and performance in the dynamic world of bodybuilding for women over forty. Women over 40 can enhance their nutritional plans to support the complexities of weight training, cardiovascular exercise, and flexibility activities by understanding the subtle interactions between nutrition and training needs. Aligning nutritional decisions with training phases and goals, from pre-workout fueling to post-workout recovery, forges a synergistic alliance that unlocks the potential for prolonged vitality, resilience, and development. Precise nutrition becomes a crucial component in the bodybuilding success story; it is a tactical ally that enables women over 40 to walk their transformational path with steadfast strength and maximum health.

Chapter 9: Recovery Nutrition and Rest Days

In the dynamic landscape of bodybuilding, recovery nutrition and strategically planned rest days emerge as indispensable components, particularly for women over 40. The interplay between intense training sessions and adequate recovery profoundly influences performance, muscle adaptation, and overall well-being. In this comprehensive guide, we delve into the intricacies of recovery nutrition, explore the importance of rest days, and provide practical insights to empower women over 40 in optimizing their recovery strategies for sustained vitality and progress.

Understanding the Significance of Recovery Nutrition

1. Muscle Repair and Protein Synthesis:

- Post-Workout Window: The immediate post-workout period is a critical window for muscle repair and protein synthesis. Consuming a combination of protein and carbohydrates during this timeframe enhances nutrient uptake, supporting the recovery process.

- Optimal Protein Intake: Adequate protein intake becomes paramount for women over 40 engaged in bodybuilding. Protein serves as the building block for muscle tissue, aiding in repair and adaptation following resistance training.

2. Glycogen Replenishment:

- Carbohydrates for Energy Stores: Intense training depletes glycogen stores, the body's primary energy source. Incorporating carbohydrates in the post-workout meal supports glycogen replenishment, ensuring sustained energy for subsequent workouts.

- Balanced Macronutrient Ratio: A balanced ratio of carbohydrates to protein in the post-workout period optimizes both muscle glycogen restoration and protein synthesis. This synergy contributes to efficient recovery.

3. Hydration for Recovery:

- Fluid Balance: Hydration is fundamental to the recovery process. Replenishing fluids lost through sweat supports overall physiological function and aids in nutrient transport to cells.

- Electrolyte Considerations: In situations involving significant fluid loss, particularly in warm environments, considering electrolyte-rich beverages or supplements enhances rehydration and maintains electrolyte balance.

4. Anti-Inflammatory Nutrition:

- Omega-3 Fatty Acids: Incorporating foods rich in omega-3 fatty acids, such as fatty fish and flaxseeds, contributes to an anti-inflammatory environment. Managing inflammation is crucial for efficient recovery and joint health, especially for women over 40.

- Colorful Fruits and Vegetables: Phytonutrients found in colorful fruits and vegetables possess anti-inflammatory properties. Including a variety of these foods supports overall health and aids in recovery.

Tailoring Recovery Nutrition to Individual Needs

1. Protein Timing and Distribution:

- Protein-Rich Snacks: Including protein-rich snacks between meals ensures a consistent supply of amino acids throughout the day. This approach supports ongoing muscle protein synthesis and aids in recovery.

- Pre-Bed Protein: Consuming a source of protein before bedtime provides a sustained release of amino acids during the overnight fasting period. This strategy supports muscle repair and minimizes the potential for muscle breakdown.

2. Individualized Macronutrient Ratios:

- Flexibility in Ratios: While general guidelines exist, individual responses to macronutrient ratios may vary. Some women over 40 may benefit from a higher carbohydrate intake post-workout, while others may find a more balanced approach effective. Personal preferences and tolerance play key roles in determining optimal ratios.

- Periodic Assessments: Regularly assessing how the body responds to different macronutrient ratios supports the refinement of recovery nutrition strategies. Adjustments based on energy levels, recovery metrics, and overall well-being contribute to individualized optimization.

3. Adaptogens for Stress Management:

- Incorporating Adaptogenic Herbs: Stress, whether physical or emotional, impacts recovery. Adaptogenic herbs like ashwagandha or rhodiola may assist in stress management, enhancing the body's ability to adapt to training stressors.

- Consistent Use for Resilience: Integrating adaptogens consistently, whether through supplementation or inclusion in teas, supports overall resilience. This becomes particularly relevant for women over 40 managing diverse responsibilities.

The Importance of Planned Rest Days

1. Muscle Repair and Adaptation:

- Essential for Growth: Rest days are not periods of inactivity but crucial intervals for muscle repair and adaptation. Giving muscles time to recover allows for optimal growth and strength gains, vital aspects of bodybuilding for women over 40.

- Prevention of Overtraining: Adequate rest prevents overtraining, a condition characterized by fatigue, decreased performance, and increased risk of injury. Overtraining can impede progress and compromise overall well-being.

2. Central Nervous System Recovery:

- CNS Fatigue Prevention: Intense training places stress on the central nervous system (CNS). Rest days prevent CNS fatigue, ensuring that the body's regulatory systems recover and function optimally.

- Improved Cognitive Function: Adequate rest contributes to improved cognitive function. Mental clarity and focus are essential for effective training sessions and overall performance.

3. Injury Prevention:

- Tissue Repair and Adaptation: The body's tissues, including muscles, ligaments, and tendons, undergo repair and adaptation during rest. This process is integral to injury prevention, particularly for women over 40 who may be more susceptible to certain injuries.

- Joint Health: Giving joints a break from repetitive stress supports joint health. This is crucial for long-term well-being, aligning with the goal of sustainable bodybuilding practices.

Strategic Nutrition on Rest Days

1. Adjusting Caloric Intake:

- Caloric Maintenance: On rest days, where energy expenditure is lower, adjusting caloric intake to maintenance levels prevents unnecessary surplus. This approach aligns with overall body composition goals.

- Prioritizing Nutrient Density: While caloric intake may decrease on rest days, prioritizing nutrient-dense foods ensures that essential vitamins and minerals are still supplied. This supports overall health and recovery.

2. Protein Emphasis for Repair:

- Slightly Increased Protein Intake: Emphasizing protein intake on rest days supports ongoing muscle repair and adaptation. While total caloric needs may be lower, maintaining protein intake helps preserve lean muscle mass.

- Distributed Protein Intake: Spreading protein intake across meals on rest days ensures a continuous supply of amino acids. This approach aligns with the goal of supporting muscle protein synthesis throughout the day.

3. Hydration Focus:

- Consistent Hydration: Maintaining consistent hydration on rest days remains essential. Hydration supports overall physiological function, aids in recovery, and contributes to general well-being.

- Herbal Teas and Hydrating Foods: Including herbal teas and hydrating foods, such as water-rich fruits and vegetables, adds variety to hydration strategies on rest days.

Mindful Recovery Practices

1. Active Recovery Strategies:

- Low-Intensity Activities: Engaging in low-intensity activities on rest days, such as walking or gentle yoga, promotes blood flow, reduces muscle stiffness, and supports overall recovery.

- Mindful Movement: Incorporating mindful movement practices fosters a connection between the body and mind. Practices like tai chi or gentle stretching enhance the recovery process.

2. Sleep Quality:

- Prioritizing Sleep on Rest Days: Rest days provide an opportunity to prioritize sleep

 duration and quality. Quality sleep is integral to hormonal balance, muscle recovery, and overall well-being.

- Consistent Sleep Patterns: Maintaining consistent sleep patterns, even on rest days, aligns with the body's circadian rhythm. This contributes to optimal recovery and adaptation.

3. Stress Reduction Techniques:

- Mindfulness and Relaxation: Incorporating mindfulness or relaxation techniques on rest days supports stress reduction. Managing stress is crucial for recovery and overall health.

- Breathing Exercises: Simple breathing exercises, practiced on rest days, contribute to relaxation and enhance parasympathetic nervous system activity, promoting a state of rest and recovery.

Individualization and Monitoring Progress

1. Listening to the Body:

- Body Signals: Paying attention to signals from the body guides recovery strategies. Sensations of fatigue, soreness, or changes in energy levels inform adjustments to training intensity, recovery nutrition, and rest day practices.

- Balancing Challenges and Adaptation: Striking a balance between challenging workouts and adequate recovery promotes adaptation. Recognizing when modifications are needed ensures sustainable progress.

2. Adapting to Lifestyle Factors:

- Flexibility in Scheduling: Adapting training schedules to accommodate lifestyle factors, such as work commitments or family responsibilities, enhances consistency. Consistency is a key factor in achieving long-term bodybuilding goals.

- Integration of Practices: Integrating recovery practices seamlessly into daily life, whether through nutrition, sleep, or stress management, supports a holistic approach to well-being.

In the journey of bodybuilding for women over 40, recovery nutrition and strategically planned rest days emerge as nurturing pillars that cultivate strength, resilience, and sustained vitality. By understanding the intricate balance between intense training, thoughtful nutrition, and mindful recovery practices, women over 40 can optimize their bodybuilding endeavors. The synergy between targeted recovery nutrition, purposeful rest days, and individualized approaches creates a harmonious foundation for achieving and surpassing fitness goals. In this tapestry of strength and well-being, the wisdom of embracing rest becomes a source of power—a vital component in the pursuit of enduring strength, vibrant health, and the realization of one's full potential.

Chapter 10: Addressing Common Challenges

In the pursuit of bodybuilding excellence for women over 40, common challenges often surface, demanding tailored solutions. Metabolic shifts, hormonal fluctuations, and potential time constraints pose obstacles that require strategic navigation. Crafting a resilient mindset becomes pivotal, embracing progress over perfection and adapting training and nutrition to individual needs. Mitigating stress through mindfulness practices supports hormonal balance, while prioritizing sleep aids in recovery. Balancing family and work commitments necessitates flexible training schedules, fostering consistency. Recognizing that the journey is unique for each woman over 40, addressing these challenges with personalized approaches ensures a sustainable path to strength, vitality, and the fulfillment of bodybuilding aspirations.

Metabolism Changes

As women transition into their 40s, metabolic changes become a prominent aspect of their bodybuilding journey. Understanding and effectively navigating these shifts are crucial for optimizing training outcomes, body composition, and overall well-being.

Metabolic Slowdown: A Natural Evolution

One notable change is the gradual metabolic slowdown that accompanies aging. The basal metabolic rate (BMR), the calories burned at rest, tends to decrease. This reduction is partly attributed to changes in body composition, including a decline in muscle mass and an increase in fat mass. As lean muscle mass plays a significant role in calorie expenditure, preserving and building muscle becomes a strategic focus for women over 40.

Hormonal Influence on Metabolism

Hormonal fluctuations further contribute to metabolic changes in this age group. The decline in estrogen during perimenopause and menopause can impact how the body stores and utilizes fat. Insulin sensitivity may decrease, affecting carbohydrate metabolism. Proactively managing these hormonal shifts through nutrition and lifestyle choices is vital for maintaining metabolic health.

Strategies for Optimizing Metabolism

1. Resistance Training Emphasis:

Prioritizing resistance training is paramount for women over 40. Engaging in regular strength training exercises helps counteract the decline in muscle mass and boosts metabolism by enhancing the body's ability to burn calories at rest. Compound exercises targeting multiple muscle groups prove particularly effective.

2. Balanced Nutrition:

Adopting a balanced and nutrient-dense diet supports metabolic health. Adequate protein intake is crucial for preserving lean muscle mass and promoting a feeling of fullness, which can aid in weight management. Including complex carbohydrates, healthy fats, and micronutrient-rich foods contributes to overall metabolic function.

3. Interval Training Incorporation:

Incorporating interval training into cardiovascular workouts proves beneficial for metabolism. High-intensity intervals elevate the heart rate and stimulate calorie burn, both during and after the workout. This approach can counteract the natural decline in calorie expenditure associated with aging.

4. Consistent Hydration:

Sufficient hydration is often underestimated in its impact on metabolism. Water is essential for various metabolic processes, including those related to energy production and nutrient transport. Women over 40 should prioritize consistent water intake throughout the day.

5. Adequate Sleep:

Quality sleep is a cornerstone of metabolic health. Sleep influences hormones that regulate appetite and energy balance. Ensuring sufficient and restful sleep supports overall well-being and aids in mitigating metabolic challenges.

6. Regular Meal Timing:

Consistent meal timing and avoiding prolonged periods of fasting contribute to metabolic stability. Spreading meals throughout the day helps regulate blood sugar levels and sustains energy levels, supporting an efficient metabolism.

7. Stress Management:

Chronic stress can negatively impact metabolism. Implementing stress management techniques, such as meditation or deep breathing exercises, is crucial. These practices contribute to hormonal balance and create an environment conducive to optimal metabolic function.

Navigating Individual Variability

It's important to recognize that individual responses to metabolic changes vary. Factors such as genetics, lifestyle, and overall health influence how a woman's metabolism evolves in her 40s. Regular self-assessment, including monitoring energy levels, sleep quality, and body composition, allows for personalized adjustments to nutrition and training strategies.

Embracing the Evolution

In essence, the metabolic changes women experience in their 40s are a natural part of the aging process. Rather than viewing these shifts as obstacles, embracing them as a facet of personal evolution can foster a positive and proactive mindset. The combination of strategic resistance training, balanced nutrition, and lifestyle adjustments empowers women over 40 to navigate these metabolic changes effectively, fostering strength, vitality, and a holistic approach to bodybuilding.

Dealing with Menopause

Menopause, a significant physiological transition for women typically occurring in their late 40s or early 50s, brings about a range of hormonal and physical changes. Successfully navigating menopause is a crucial aspect of the bodybuilding journey for women over 40. Understanding the challenges posed by hormonal shifts and adopting a comprehensive approach can empower women to continue their bodybuilding endeavors with resilience and vitality.

Hormonal Dynamics During Menopause

Menopause is marked by the cessation of menstrual cycles, signaling the end of reproductive years. The hormonal landscape undergoes substantial changes, with a significant decline in estrogen levels. This hormonal shift contributes to various challenges, including changes in body composition, metabolism, and bone density.

Body Composition Challenges

1. Increased Body Fat:

The decline in estrogen is associated with an increase in visceral fat, particularly around the abdominal area. This shift in fat distribution can pose challenges for women over 40 in their bodybuilding pursuits, affecting both aesthetics and health.

2. Loss of Lean Muscle Mass:

Estrogen plays a role in maintaining muscle mass, and its reduction during menopause can lead to a decline in lean muscle. Preserving and building muscle becomes a strategic focus to counteract this natural loss.

Metabolic Considerations

1. Metabolic Rate Changes:

The decrease in estrogen levels can contribute to a decline in metabolic rate. This shift may necessitate adjustments to caloric intake and expenditure to maintain body composition and overall metabolic health.

2. Insulin Sensitivity Challenges:

Menopause can also impact insulin sensitivity, influencing how the body processes carbohydrates. Managing carbohydrate intake and choosing complex carbohydrates become crucial for metabolic stability.

Bone Health Implications

1. Bone Density Reduction:

Estrogen plays a key role in maintaining bone density. The hormonal changes during menopause increase the risk of bone density reduction, leading to conditions like osteoporosis. Incorporating bone-strengthening exercises and sufficient calcium and vitamin D intake is essential.

Comprehensive Strategies for Bodybuilding During Menopause

1. Targeted Resistance Training:

Prioritizing resistance training becomes even more critical during menopause. Progressive and targeted resistance exercises support muscle preservation and development. Compound movements, such as squats and deadlifts, engage multiple muscle groups and contribute to overall strength.

2. Optimized Nutrition:

Adapting nutritional strategies is pivotal. Ensuring an adequate intake of protein, especially leucine-rich sources, supports muscle protein synthesis. Additionally, incorporating foods rich in calcium and vitamin D aids in preserving bone health.

3. Hormone Replacement Therapy (HRT) Consideration:

For some women, Hormone Replacement Therapy (HRT) may be a consideration under the guidance of healthcare professionals. HRT can help manage symptoms associated with hormonal changes, potentially supporting aspects of body composition and metabolic health.

4. Cardiovascular Exercise for Metabolism:

Incorporating cardiovascular exercises, such as interval training and aerobic activities, supports metabolic health. These exercises contribute to calorie burn and cardiovascular fitness, crucial for overall well-being during menopause.

5. Stress Management Practices:

Managing stress is paramount. Chronic stress can exacerbate hormonal imbalances and impact body composition. Practices like yoga, meditation, or mindfulness can be effective tools for stress reduction.

6. Adequate Sleep:

Quality sleep is essential for hormonal balance and overall health. Establishing consistent sleep patterns and creating a conducive sleep environment supports the body's recovery and adaptation processes.

Individualization and Patience

Recognizing the individual nature of menopausal experiences is crucial. Each woman may navigate this phase differently, and personalized approaches to training, nutrition, and lifestyle adjustments are key. Patience and a positive mindset are essential components as women over 40 adapt to and embrace the changes associated with menopause.

Navigating menopause as a woman over 40 in bodybuilding is not without its challenges, but it also presents an opportunity for empowerment and transformation. Embracing the evolving needs of the body, adopting proactive health measures, and celebrating the strength that comes with experience can redefine the bodybuilding journey during this phase of life. Through targeted strategies, resilience, and a holistic approach, women over 40 can continue to sculpt their bodies, foster vitality, and embrace the unique power that comes with navigating menopause.

Managing Stress

Stress management holds pivotal significance in the bodybuilding journey for women over 40. Beyond the physical demands of training, the intricate interplay between stress and the body's response becomes a critical factor influencing overall well-being, progress, and the attainment of fitness goals.

Understanding Stress Dynamics

Stress, whether physical or psychological, triggers the release of hormones such as cortisol and adrenaline. While these hormones are essential for the body's fight-or-flight response, chronic elevation can lead to detrimental effects. For women over 40, who may already be navigating hormonal changes, effective stress management becomes paramount.

Impact of Stress on Body Composition

1. Cortisol and Fat Storage:

Chronically elevated cortisol levels, often associated with prolonged stress, can contribute to increased abdominal fat storage. For women over 40 striving for optimal body composition, mitigating stress is crucial in preventing unwanted changes in fat distribution.

2. Muscle Breakdown:

High cortisol levels may also lead to muscle breakdown. Preserving lean muscle mass is a key goal in bodybuilding, and stress-induced muscle catabolism can hinder progress. Strategic stress management becomes a proactive measure for maintaining muscle integrity.

Strategies for Effective Stress Management

1. Mindfulness and Meditation:

Incorporating mindfulness practices, such as meditation and deep breathing exercises, offers a powerful antidote to stress. These techniques promote relaxation, reduce cortisol levels, and enhance overall emotional well-being.

2. Regular Exercise:

While intense workouts contribute to physical stress, regular exercise has a paradoxical effect on stress management. Engaging in moderate, consistent physical activity helps regulate cortisol levels, improve mood through endorphin release, and fosters a sense of accomplishment.

3. Adequate Sleep:

Quality sleep is a cornerstone of stress resilience. Establishing consistent sleep patterns and creating a conducive sleep environment support hormonal balance, cognitive function, and emotional well-being.

4. Social Support Networks:

Cultivating strong social support networks provides emotional outlets. Connecting with friends, family, or fellow fitness enthusiasts creates a sense of community, buffering against the negative impact of stress.

5. Time Management and Prioritization:

Effectively managing time and prioritizing tasks are key components of stress reduction. Women over 40 juggling multiple responsibilities benefit from setting realistic goals, breaking tasks into manageable steps, and acknowledging achievements.

6. Holistic Nutrition:

Nutrition plays a vital role in stress management. Consuming a balanced diet rich in whole foods ensures a steady supply of nutrients that support the body's stress response. Avoiding excessive caffeine and sugar, which can contribute to stress, is also prudent.

Tailoring Stress Management to Individual Needs

Recognizing that stress management is a highly individualized process is crucial. What works for one woman may not be as effective for another. Tailoring stress management strategies to individual preferences, lifestyle, and personality types enhances adherence and effectiveness.

Integrating Stress Management into Training

1. Mindful Workouts:

Infusing mindfulness into workouts enhances stress management. Focusing on the present moment during exercises, paying attention to body sensations, and embracing the mind-body connection create a holistic training experience.

2. Varied Training Intensity:

Strategically varying training intensity can mitigate overall stress on the body. Incorporating periods of lower-intensity activities, such as yoga or mobility work, provides a reprieve from high-impact training and promotes recovery.

Consistency and Long-Term Well-Being

Consistency in stress management practices contributes to long-term well-being. Stress is an inevitable part of life, but building resilience and adopting proactive measures ensure that its impact is mitigated. For women over 40 engaged in bodybuilding, stress management becomes not just a complement to training but an integral component of a holistic approach to health and fitness.

Conclusion: Empowering the Mind and Body

In the intricate tapestry of bodybuilding for women over 40, effective stress management emerges as a potent tool for empowerment. Balancing the demands of physical training with mindful stress reduction practices creates a harmonious synergy that fosters resilience, vitality, and sustainable progress. By acknowledging the interconnectedness of stress, hormones, and overall well-being, women over 40 can cultivate a powerful mindset that transcends the gym, influencing every facet of their lives. In the pursuit of strength and holistic health, mastering the art of stress management becomes a transformative journey—an investment in the enduring well-being of both the mind and the body.

Chapter 11: Creating a Sustainable and Enjoyable Diet

Crafting a diet that is both sustainable and enjoyable is a cornerstone in the bodybuilding journey for women over 40. This pivotal aspect not only influences physical well-being but also contributes significantly to overall health, energy levels, and the ability to sustain long-term fitness goals. In this comprehensive guide, we delve into the key principles and strategies for creating a diet that aligns with the unique needs of women over 40, ensuring sustainability, enjoyment, and optimal support for bodybuilding endeavors.

Understanding the Unique Needs of Women Over 40

1. Metabolic Changes:

As women age, metabolic changes, including a gradual decrease in basal metabolic rate (BMR), become more pronounced. This emphasizes the importance of tailoring dietary choices to support metabolic health and prevent unwanted changes in body composition.

2. Hormonal Influences:

Hormonal fluctuations, particularly during perimenopause and menopause, add complexity to dietary considerations. Managing these hormonal shifts through nutrition becomes integral to overall well-being.

3. Nutrient Requirements:

Meeting nutrient requirements becomes crucial for maintaining bone health, preserving lean muscle mass, and supporting the body's ability to recover from physical stress. Adequate protein, calcium, and vitamins are paramount.

Principles for Crafting a Sustainable Diet

1. Balance and Moderation:

Embracing a balanced approach involves incorporating a variety of foods in moderation. Avoiding extreme diets promotes a sustainable relationship with food, ensuring the inclusion of essential nutrients from various sources.

2. Whole Foods Emphasis:

Prioritizing whole, minimally processed foods provides a spectrum of essential nutrients. These foods contribute not only to physical health but also enhance the enjoyment of meals through diverse flavors and textures.

3. Personalized Macronutrient Ratios:

Recognizing that individuals may respond differently to macronutrient ratios allows for personalization. While protein intake is crucial for muscle health, the distribution of fats and carbohydrates can be tailored based on individual preferences and metabolic responses.

4. Flexibility and Adaptability:

Building flexibility into the diet allows for adaptability to different situations and preferences. This flexibility contributes to the sustainability of the diet over the long term, accommodating social events, travel, and varying energy needs.

Strategies for Enhancing Enjoyment in the Diet

1. Culinary Exploration:

Embracing culinary exploration adds an element of enjoyment to the diet. Trying new recipes, experimenting with different cooking techniques, and incorporating a variety of herbs and spices enhance the sensory experience of meals.

2. Mindful Eating Practices:

Engaging in mindful eating practices fosters a deeper connection with food. Paying attention to the flavors, textures, and overall dining experience promotes satisfaction and prevents mindless overeating.

3. Incorporating Cultural and Personal Favorites:

Including cultural and personal favorites in the diet creates a sense of familiarity and enjoyment. Finding ways to make traditional dishes more nutritionally aligned ensures that dietary choices resonate with personal preferences.

4. Regular but Controlled Indulgences:

Allowing for occasional indulgences contributes to diet enjoyment. Planning and savoring controlled indulgences prevent feelings of deprivation and promote a healthy relationship with treats.

Balancing Macronutrients for Optimal Health

1. Protein:

Protein intake is a foundational element, especially for women over 40 engaged in bodybuilding. Adequate protein supports muscle preservation, repair, and overall metabolic health.

2. Carbohydrates:

Tailoring carbohydrate intake to individual energy needs and preferences is crucial. Complex carbohydrates from whole grains, fruits, and vegetables provide sustained energy and essential nutrients.

3. Fats:

Including healthy fats, such as those from avocados, nuts, and olive oil, contributes to satiety and supports hormonal health. Balancing the intake of omega-3 and omega-6 fatty acids promotes overall well-being.

Micronutrient-Rich Diet: Supporting Overall Health

1. Nutrient Diversity:

Prioritizing a diet rich in micronutrients ensures comprehensive support for overall health. A colorful array of fruits and vegetables provides essential vitamins and minerals, contributing to optimal physiological function.

2. Supplementation as Needed:

Based on individual dietary patterns and needs, considering targeted micronutrient supplementation ensures potential gaps are addressed. This contributes to overall well-being and supports bodybuilding goals.

Hydration: Foundation for Vitality and Performance

1. Consistent Fluid Intake:

Maintaining consistent hydration throughout the day supports overall health and aids in cognitive function. Women over 40 should prioritize regular fluid intake, considering individual needs and activity levels.

2. Hydrating with Whole Foods:

Incorporating hydrating foods, such as water-rich fruits and vegetables, contributes to overall fluid balance. This aligns with the goal of maintaining hydration beyond traditional beverage sources.

Adapting Nutrition to Training Phases and Goals

1. Bulking and Muscle Building:

During bulking phases, adopting a slight caloric surplus supports the increased energy demands of intense resistance training. Prioritizing protein intake remains crucial, providing necessary amino acids for muscle synthesis and repair.

2. Cutting and Fat Loss:

Creating a modest caloric deficit during cutting phases supports the goal of reducing body fat. Adjusting overall caloric intake while maintaining protein intake helps preserve lean muscle mass.

3. Maintenance Phases:

Aligning caloric intake with energy expenditure during maintenance phases supports overall health. Prioritizing nutrient-dense foods ensures the body receives essential vitamins and minerals.

Individualization and Regular Assessments

1. Individualized Approach:

Tailoring nutritional strategies to individual preferences and tolerances enhances adherence. Considering factors like food preferences, dietary restrictions, and digestion aids in creating sustainable dietary plans.

2. Regular Assessments:

Monitoring performance metrics, such as strength gains and workout endurance, provides insights into the effectiveness of nutrition in supporting training intensity. Assessing recovery, including muscle soreness and fatigue, informs adjustments to nutritional strategies.

Lifestyle Factors and Consistency
1. Sleep Quality:

Prioritizing quality sleep is integral to supporting recovery from intense training sessions. Ensuring adequate and restful sleep contributes to hormonal balance, cognitive function, and overall well-being.

2. Stress Management:

Effective stress management complements dietary efforts. Chronic stress can impact hormonal balance and metabolism, highlighting the interconnectedness of lifestyle factors in achieving bodybuilding goals.

3. Consistency Over Time:

Consistency over time is the linchpin of success. Sustainable and enjoyable dietary choices, coupled with lifestyle factors, create a foundation for long-term adherence and progress in the bodybuilding journey.

In the intricate dance of bodybuilding for women over 40, crafting a sustainable and enjoyable diet emerges as both an art and a science. This holistic approach transcends mere nutrition—it becomes a celebration of the body's strength, a harmonious journey of flavors and textures, and a profound investment in enduring well-being. By weaving together the threads of balance, enjoyment, and individualization, women over 40 can not only achieve their bodybuilding goals but also savor the journey, nurturing both body and spirit along the path to enduring vitality.

Conclusion

In the vibrant tapestry of bodybuilding for women over 40, the journey extends far beyond lifting weights and sculpting muscles—it is an exploration of strength, wellness, and joy. Crafting a sustainable and enjoyable diet stands as a cornerstone, intertwining with the intricacies of metabolism, hormonal shifts, and the evolving needs of the body. The principles of balance, moderation, and whole-food emphasis create a canvas upon which the artistry of nutrition unfolds.

As women navigate the unique challenges of metabolic changes and hormonal transitions, the wisdom of personalization becomes evident. Flexibility in macronutrient ratios, mindful eating practices, and the infusion of culinary exploration enrich the experience, making every meal a celebration of nourishment.

The dynamic interplay between nutrition and training phases underscores the adaptability required in the pursuit of diverse goals. From bulking and muscle building to cutting and fat loss, and through maintenance phases, the diet becomes a fluid companion, adjusting to the ever-changing landscape of fitness aspirations.

Hydration, often underestimated, flows as a foundation for vitality and performance. Consistent fluid intake, complemented by hydrating whole foods, sustains the body's resilience through intense workouts and recovery phases.

Yet, beyond the realm of macros and micros, the essence of this journey lies in individualization and regular assessments. Recognizing the uniqueness of each woman's body and regularly assessing its responses not only refines nutritional strategies but also deepens the connection between mind and body.

In the broader context of lifestyle factors, the importance of quality sleep and effective stress management emerges. These elements, woven into the fabric of daily life, amplify the impact of nutrition on hormonal balance, recovery, and overall well-being.

Consistency over time emerges as the guiding force—an unwavering commitment to the principles of a sustainable and enjoyable diet. Through the ebb and flow of training phases, the evolving needs of the body, and the tapestry of personal preferences, consistency becomes the brushstroke that paints the masterpiece of enduring wellness.

As women over 40 embrace this holistic approach to bodybuilding, they embark on a journey of self-discovery and empowerment. It's not merely about the sets and reps, the calories and macros; it's about nurturing the body, savoring the flavors of a well-crafted diet, and finding joy in the strength that unfolds with each passing day.

In conclusion, the art of bodybuilding for women over 40 is a celebration—a celebration of strength, wellness, and the joy that arises from harmonizing the body's needs with the pleasures of nourishment. Through the synergy of balanced nutrition, tailored training, and a commitment to holistic well-being, women over 40 not only build their bodies but also cultivate a profound sense of vitality that resonates in every aspect of their lives. As the journey unfolds, may it be adorned with strength, wellness, and the sheer joy of embracing the remarkable power within.

CONTACT US

FREE 30 DAYS MEAL PLANNER

FREE 30Days Meal Planner, a priceless extra to get you started on the path to a more organized and healthy living. This meticulously curated planner is made to make meal planning easier, save you time, and help you meet your nutritional objectives. Having a month's worth of recipes makes it simpler than ever to stick to your diet goals. Prepare to enjoy the advantages of this wonderful resource! Scan the QR Code below now.